To Sherry + Alvin,
much love
Sol

Many Good Wishes and
Best of luck Always
Jane Conway Caske

The Nantucket Diet™

*A Safe and Effective 3-Phase Program
for Permanent Weight Loss
and a Healthy Lifestyle*

SOL JACOBS, M.D.
and
JANE CONWAY CASPE

BALLANTINE BOOKS • NEW YORK

A Ballantine Book
Published by The Random House Publishing Group

Copyright © 2005 by Sol Jacobs, M.D., and Jane Conway Caspe

www.ballantinebooks.com

LIBRARY OF CONGRESS CATALOGING-IN-PUBLICATION DATA

Jacobs, Sol.
   The Nantucket diet : [a safe and effective 3-phase program for permanent weight loss and a healthy lifestyle] / by Sol Jacobs and Jane Conway Caspe.—1st ed.
     p. cm.
   Includes index.
   ISBN 0-345-47677-8
   1. Reducing diets.   I. Caspe, Jane Conway.   II. Title.

RM222.2J3124 2005
613.2'5—dc22   2004052549

Text design by Susan Turner

Manufactured in the United States of America

First Edition: June 2005

1 3 5 7 9 8 6 4 2

We dedicate this book to our parents:

My mom, Alexandra Conway, is my best friend and the woman that I admire most in this world. She continues to fill my life with love, laughter, and happiness. My dad, Paul Conway, a Nantucket native, passed away several years ago. He was always there for me, taught me the value of living, and instilled a love and appreciation for Nantucket that remains in my heart today. They always thought that they could have been better parents, but there is no better than best.

Norma Glazer Jacobs, who was a woman of great courage and integrity and a talented musician, and Julian Jacobs, a friend and a role model as father and physician.

FOREWORD BY MICHAEL ROSENBLATT, M.D.

Our nation is facing a health crisis as our families, friends, and neighbors fall victim at ever younger ages to complications of obesity such as diabetes and heart disease. Our health care system is not prepared for the widening epidemic of obesity and metabolic syndrome.

Healthy lifestyle and diet are the most promising components of the solution to the epidemic. But fad diets continue to sidetrack the medical community's best efforts to teach lifestyle modification for weight loss. Calorie restriction and exercise aren't being successfully "marketed" to the general public. As Dr. Jacobs points out, the very fact that fad diets have been widely embraced as the number of overweight and obese Americans increases is in and of itself evidence that such diets are not the solution. The public deserves to hear the truth about weight gain and loss. Poor diets and sedentary lifestyles need to change. Dramatic dietary changes are not maintainable; if a diet is not maintainable, it cannot succeed. Energy balance is a rule of physics. This rule applies to all of us although each of us would love to convince ourselves and our doctors otherwise.

The Nantucket Diet is a credible weight-loss guide and resource for the general public. It is a clearly written, well-referenced and scientifically validated approach to weight loss. The weight loss recommendations are supported by the scientific literature and are in line with current national weight-loss guidelines. This book's clear and innovative use of energy expenditure provides an understanding of and solution to weight problems. Dr. Jacobs also provides a provocative look at the history, science, and politics of obesity, discusses the connection of the insulin resistance syndrome to heart disease, and notes the critical role food choices play in this regard. Behavioral modification is reviewed. The interplay of carbohydrates, glycemic index, and insulin levels is explained from the vantage point of an endocrinologist.

Since *The Nantucket Diet* manuscript was submitted for publication there have been two noteworthy developments. The 2005 Federal

Dietary Guidelines were revealed in August 2004 and the recommendations are consistent with the philosophy of this book. It is calorie restriction that determines weight loss, not the percentage of carbohydrate, fat
or protein intake. The glycemic index "is of little utility" for weight loss.
Exercise is important.* In addition, Medicare revised its obesity coverage policy removing language that at one time did not classify obesity as
a medical condition.† This direction in public policy also supports the
message of this book and helps direct attention (and hopefully funds) to
the management of obesity.

Each spring, medical school seniors become doctors and face the
medical consequences of overweight and obesity. Whether they become
primary care providers, medical subspecialists or surgeons, obesity will
have an impact on their practice of medicine. These young doctors will
need to respond to the call to action that Dr. Jacobs reviews in Chapter 1 and practice the lifestyle that they preach. One of our jobs as edu-
cators is to teach them to provide comprehensive and compassionate
care to the ever-growing population of overweight patients and avoid
the pitfalls of physician bias. I hope that guidance from books like *The
Nantucket Diet* will lead to better-informed patients and help make
patient encounters with physicians more productive. In the meantime,
the cutting edge basic science and clinical research on obesity at Tufts
University School of Medicine and other institutions across the country
will continue, more needed than ever before.

MICHAEL ROSENBLATT, M.D.
Dean, Tufts University School of Medicine
Professor of Physiology and Medicine,
Tufts University School of Medicine

---

* www.health.gov/dietaryguidelines/dga2005/report; October 25, 2004.
† www.omhrc.gov/OMHRC/pressreleases/2004press0715a.htm; October 25, 2004.

ACKNOWLEDGMENTS

Thank you to my partner and coauthor Dr. Sol Jacobs for his incredible commitment, dedication, and friendship throughout this whole process. Thank you to my partner and brother Dr. Laurence Conway for being by my side with love and support my whole life.

I would like to thank my husband Mitch for his constant love and encouragement during my work on this book and every day of our lives together.

Lastly, I would like to acknowledge my nephew Alex, my stepson Scott, and my niece Gabrielle. Seeing Nantucket through their eyes reminds me of how important the island is to my whole family.

Thanks to my wife Karen for her unconditional love, companionship, and support.

Thanks to Jane Conway Caspe. I am indebted to Jane for her enthusiasm, hard work, and friendship.

We would like to thank Dan Menaker for making this book possible.

Thanks to Maureen O'Neal, Johanna Bowman, Caroline Sutton, Christina Duffy, and the superb team at Random House.

Thank you to Maureen Callahan, Dr. Michael Rosenblatt, Sue Warga, Josh Karpf, Ron Minsk, Cindy Murray, Sarah Glazer, Fred Nowicki, Lenore Jacobs, Marianne Nowicki, Dr. Harold Goldstein, Dr. Richard Siegel, Dr. David Blaustein, Joyce McCarthy, Theodore MacVeagh, Steve Mintz, Laura Goldin, Dominique Mallette, Jody Lou Lifton, Clark Evans, Jane MacDonald, the Nantucket Chamber of Commerce, the Town of Nantucket, Nantucket Vineyards, and Nantucket Nectars, as well as all of the restaurants and family members who contributed recipes to our book.

CONTENTS

INTRODUCTION

Residents of and visitors to modern-day Nantucket enjoy its invigorating outdoor lifestyle, charming New England character, and picturesque landscapes that are the heritage of the island's seafaring days of old. Nantucket's culinary culture, with its celebrated gourmet recipes from the sea, provides the final bit of distinction to a "faraway land" of living history, maritime mystique, and cultural refinement.

Exercise on the island, however, was not always an activity of leisure. Nantucket's physically fit whalers of past generations routinely balanced their calorie intake with very demanding labor. This vigorous physical activity, which was the definition of a hard day's work at sea, and the hearty traditional diet that has been part and parcel of life on Nantucket through her modern history, inspired the title and message of this book. Weight gain or loss is as straightforward as the balance between calorie intake and energy expenditure. This is a fact of life for us today, just as it was for these sailors, and admitting this to ourselves is the first step to successful weight loss.

We are confident that you will find *The Nantucket Diet* a valuable resource for living a healthier life, and in an era of conflicting dietary advice, a refreshing way to focus on a sensible and effective path to weight loss. Our weight-loss recommendations are evidence-based and in line with currently accepted national dietary guidelines. The changes we propose are effective, maintainable and, most important, adaptable to your individual needs.

In addition to exploring the impact that overweight and obesity are having on our nation's health, we address the general principles of nutrition and weight loss as they apply to your health and explain why the fad diets you've tried in the past don't work. *The Nantucket Diet* provides a scientifically sound alternative to the drastic dietary changes, repeated frustration, and weight regain of popular diets that feed off the American quick-fix psyche. This is not another fad diet.

Should you choose to follow our diet program to the letter to achieve sustained weight loss, or apply its general principles toward a healthier diet, you will be able to use the information found in the following pages as a guide to improved fitness and an enhanced sense of well-being. We know you will also enjoy the wonderful recipes from many of the premier restaurants on the island of Nantucket.

Sol Jacobs, M.D.

Jane Conway Caspe

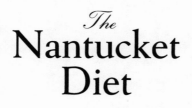

The
Nantucket
Diet

Chapter 1

The Origins, Science, and Politics of Weight Gain

The human body has evolved to store excess calories. Our ancestors lived in an environment that was harsh and unpredictable. Food was a precious commodity not easily obtained. The majority of calories were gathered by women carrying children on their hips, while men would occasionally come home with the spoils of a hunt. Families were constantly on the move, living in small groups so that their demand for calories did not outstrip the supply.[1] Our hunter-gatherer ancestors stored calories as fat in times of relative food surplus and then burned these stored calories during the inevitable times of food shortage. These food shortages could occur as often as several times per year, as plants and wild game were frequently scarce and many groups were competing for the same resources. Gaining weight during times of food surplus was an evolutionary advantage in this environment, a very specific environment that no longer exists.[2]

We are therefore attempting to defy our genetic inheritance. Our bodies, programmed over hundreds of thousands of years to store excess calories as fat, have been thrown into the industrialized world, where food is high in calories and easily obtained in absurd abundance 365 days per year. We eat far more calories than we need to survive and reproduce (our evolutionary purpose), and our bodies store these calories as fat to be burned during a time of food shortage that will never come. It is not that our bodies are defective—they are doing the job they have evolved to do. Unfortunately, there is no current need for this specific ability. It has been suggested that economic success in our market economy encourages less exercise and more eating.[3] As we have become more sedentary and our diets have become higher in calories, we as a society have failed to burn our excess calories. As a result, obesity and overweight have become epidemic in the Western world. Certainly genetics plays a role in the development of obesity, and some people will have a harder time losing weight than others, but no one doubts that environment plays a role even across this genetic variation.

While we may live more comfortable lives than our ancestors, the resulting obesity and overweight (to be defined shortly) carry with them the risk of multiple health problems and premature death. For many years healthy weight range determinations were based partly on data collected by life insurance companies in the late 1950s. Since that time multiple studies have shown an association between excess weight gain and risk of death.[4]

Unfortunately, in spite of a now growing appreciation for the risks of obesity both by the general public and by physicians, the obesity problem in this country has dramatically worsened over the last decade. We are facing an epidemic in the true sense of the word. The World Health Organization has declared obesity one of the top health dangers to the developed world.[5] This not only is a problem for the adult population but is increasingly affecting our teens and children. As a result, diseases such as type 2 diabetes (ironically previously known as adult-onset diabetes) occur now with startling frequency in progressively younger patients. Up to 33 percent of diabetes diagnosed in childhood turned out to be type 2 diabetes according to a 1996 report.[6]

How are obesity and overweight defined? Traditionally, men with more than 25 percent body fat or women with more than 35 percent body fat have been considered obese.[7] Clinicians now, however, use a measurement called the body mass index (BMI) as a good indirect estimate of a person's percentage of body fat. While the BMI is quite good at estimating the percentage of body fat in most individuals, it is less accurate in bodybuilders, who have a higher percentage of muscle for any given weight; in them the BMI overestimates the percentage of body fat. The BMI is also likely less accurate in the elderly, who have less lean body mass; in them the measure underestimates the percentage of body fat. Use the charts on pages 6 and 7 to determine your BMI and to estimate your percentage of body fat. You can also go to the Nantucket Diet's Web site (www.nantucketdiet.com) to quickly determine your BMI using the BMI calculator.

Calculating the BMI allows a clinician to conveniently chart a continuum of increasing health risk as a person's weight (and percentage of body fat) increases. Evidence from large studies of both men and women show increased risk of diabetes, high blood pressure, and heart disease as BMI increases. The risk of other diseases such as arthritis, stroke, sleep apnea, colon cancer, endometrial cancer, postmenopausal breast cancer, and infertility also rises with increasing BMI.[8] Thus individuals who lose weight will likely decrease their risk of disease and death as their BMI drops.

In addition to BMI, it is well established that an individual's physical distribution of excess weight is related to heart disease risk. A pattern of obesity in which most excess fat is gained in the abdominal cavity, termed central obesity, leads to the insulin resistance syndrome (high blood pressure, abnormal cholesterol levels, diabetes, and coagulation and blood vessel wall abnormalities) and results in a particularly high incidence of cardiovascular disease such as heart attack and stroke. Therefore, even for the same BMI, heart disease risk is increased when more weight is gained as fat around the abdomen in the so called central pattern. The table on page 8 lists relative heart disease risk based on waist measurement even within the same BMI categories.[9]

In June 1998 the National Institutes of Health published its "Clinical Guidelines on the Identification, Evaluation and Treatment of Obesity." The expert panel that prepared these guidelines suggested that, given population studies showing an increased risk of death in individuals with a BMI over 25 and particularly a BMI over 30 (as much as a 100 percent increased risk of death from heart disease), the BMI cutoff values of 25 and 30 should be considered the clinical definitions of overweight and obesity, respectively.[10] Therefore, to health care providers, the terms *overweight* and *obesity* should have specific medical definitions and not simply be colloquialisms or slang terms. It follows that health care providers should base their diagnosis and treatment of obesity accordingly.

BMI

Find your height in inches on the left (5 feet = 60 inches) and then follow to the right to find your weight in pounds. Your BMI will be at the top of the chart directly above your weight.

BODY MASS INDEX TABLE

Height (Inches)	Normal						Overweight					Obese										Extreme Obesity														
BMI	19	20	21	22	23	24	25	26	27	28	29	30	31	32	33	34	35	36	37	38	39	40	41	42	43	44	45	46	47	48	49	50	51	52	53	54
												Body Weight (pounds)																								
58	91	96	100	105	110	115	119	124	129	134	138	143	148	153	158	162	167	172	177	181	186	191	196	201	205	210	215	220	224	229	234	239	244	248	253	258
59	94	99	104	109	114	119	124	128	133	138	143	148	153	158	163	168	173	178	183	188	193	198	203	208	212	217	222	227	232	237	242	247	252	257	262	267
60	97	102	107	112	118	123	128	133	138	143	148	153	158	163	168	174	179	184	189	194	199	204	209	215	220	225	230	235	240	245	250	255	261	266	271	276
61	100	106	111	116	122	127	132	137	143	148	153	158	164	169	174	180	185	190	195	201	206	211	217	222	227	232	238	243	248	254	259	264	269	275	280	285
62	104	109	115	120	126	131	136	142	147	153	158	164	169	175	180	186	191	196	202	207	213	218	224	229	235	240	246	251	256	262	267	273	278	284	289	295
63	107	113	118	124	130	135	141	146	152	158	163	169	175	180	186	191	197	203	208	214	220	225	231	237	242	248	254	259	265	270	278	282	287	293	299	304
64	110	116	122	128	134	140	145	151	157	163	169	174	180	186	192	197	204	209	215	221	227	232	238	244	250	256	262	267	273	279	285	291	296	302	308	314
65	114	120	126	132	138	144	150	156	162	168	174	180	186	192	198	204	210	216	222	228	234	240	246	252	258	264	270	276	282	288	294	300	306	312	318	324
66	118	124	130	136	142	148	155	161	167	173	179	186	192	198	204	210	216	223	229	235	241	247	253	260	266	272	278	284	291	297	303	309	315	322	328	334
67	121	127	134	140	146	153	159	166	172	178	185	191	198	204	211	217	223	230	236	242	249	255	261	268	274	280	287	293	299	306	312	319	325	331	338	344
68	125	131	138	144	151	158	164	171	177	184	190	197	203	210	216	223	230	236	243	249	256	262	269	276	282	289	295	302	308	315	322	328	335	341	348	354
69	128	135	142	149	155	162	169	176	182	189	196	203	209	216	223	230	236	243	250	257	263	270	277	284	291	297	304	311	318	324	331	338	345	351	358	365
70	132	139	146	153	160	167	174	181	188	195	202	209	216	222	229	236	243	250	257	264	271	278	285	292	299	306	313	320	327	334	341	348	355	362	369	376
71	136	143	150	157	165	172	179	186	193	200	208	215	222	229	236	243	250	257	265	272	279	286	293	301	308	315	322	329	338	343	351	358	365	372	379	386
72	140	147	154	162	169	177	184	191	199	206	213	221	228	235	242	250	258	265	272	279	287	294	302	309	316	324	331	338	346	353	361	368	375	383	390	397
73	144	151	159	166	174	182	189	197	204	212	219	227	235	242	250	257	265	272	280	288	295	302	310	318	325	333	340	348	355	363	371	378	386	393	401	408
74	148	155	163	171	179	186	194	202	210	218	225	233	241	249	256	264	272	280	287	295	303	311	319	326	334	342	350	358	365	373	381	389	396	404	412	420
75	152	160	168	176	184	192	200	208	216	224	232	240	248	256	264	272	279	287	295	303	311	319	327	335	343	351	359	367	375	383	391	399	407	415	423	431
76	156	164	172	180	189	197	205	213	221	230	238	246	254	263	271	279	287	295	304	312	320	328	336	344	353	361	369	377	385	394	402	410	418	426	435	443

Reproduced from National Heart, Lung, and Blood Institute Web document "Clinical Guidelines on the Identification, Evaluation and Treatment of Overweight & Obesity in Adults" (www.nhlbi.nih.gov/guidelines/obesity/bmi_tbl.pdf)

PERCENTAGE BODY FAT BASED ON BMI IN MEN

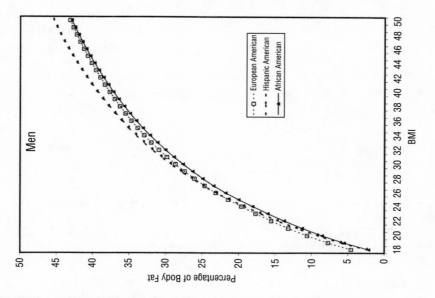

Adapted from Hernandez, J et al; The American Journal of Clinical Nutrition Vol. 77, No 1, 71–75, January 2003.
Reproduced with permission by the American Journal of Clinical Nutrition. © Am J Clin Nutr. American Society for Clinical Nutrition

PERCENTAGE BODY FAT BASED ON BMI IN WOMEN

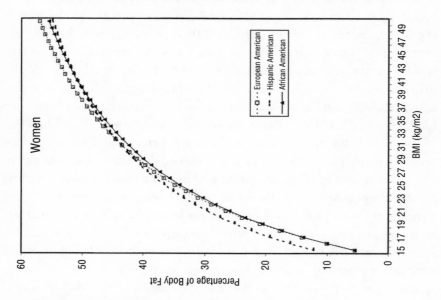

Adapted from Hernandez, J. et al; The American Journal of Clinical Nutrition Vol. 77, No 1, 71–75, January 2003.
Reproduced with permission by the American Journal of Clinical Nutrition. © Am J Clin Nutr. American Society for Clinical Nutrition.

CLASSIFICATION OF OVERWEIGHT AND OBESITY BY BMI, WAIST CIRCUMFERENCE, AND ASSOCIATED DISEASE RISKS

	BMI	Obesity Class	DISEASE RISK RELATIVE TO NORMAL WEIGHT AND WAIST CIRCUMFERENCE Men ≤ 40 in Women ≤ 35 in	> 40 in > 35 in
Underweight	<18.5		—	—
Normal	18.5–24.9		—	—
Overweight	25.0–29.9		Increased	High
Obesity	30.0–34.9	I	High	Very High
	35.0–39.9	II	Very High	Very High
Extreme Obesity	≥40	III	Extremely High	Extremely High

Adapted from National Heart, Lung, and Blood Institute Web document "Clinical Guidelines on the Identification, Evaluation, and Treatment of Overweight & Obesity in Adults: Executive Summary" (www.nhlbi.gov/guidelines/obesity/sum_clin.htm)

Recent data have demonstrated that 65 percent of the United States adult population meets the above-mentioned BMI-based definition of overweight while the prevalence of obesity in adult Americans is estimated at 30 percent.[11] The prevalence of severe obesity has quadrupled to one in fifty adult Americans in the past fifteen years.[12] It is estimated that 39 percent of U.S. adults will be obese by 2008.[13] The numbers regarding children are just as alarming. Up to 15 percent of children in the United States are overweight, and this number approaches 25 percent for minorities such as African Americans and Hispanics.[14] Unfortunately, weight gain among children is also occurring in other developed areas of the world. A recent study in Australia revealed that the percentage of children ages seven to fifteen who are overweight or obese doubled from 1985 to 1997. Excessive weight is truly a global problem.[15]

As noted above, overweight and obese American adults and children face a higher risk of cardiovascular disease, diabetes, cancer of many types, and a host of other weight-related health problems such as arthritis and sleep apnea. Data published in 2003 suggest that severe obesity in relatively young adults will result in the loss of between eight and thirteen years of life, potentially representing up to a 22 percent reduction in their remaining years.[16] These are years lost with their loved ones and productive years lost to society—an immeasurable toll. In fact, obesity is now the number two preventable cause of death in the United States, second only to smoking, currently resulting in as many as 400,000 deaths per year.[17] The financial cost of obesity is also staggering. Obesity and its resulting health problems cost us $99 billion per year, approximately half of which is direct medical costs.[18]

It should also be pointed out that the cost of obesity is not measured only in disease or health care dollars. There is considerable bias against and discrimination toward overweight and obese individuals, and they may therefore incur a significant psychological toll as a result of the insensitive attitudes held by society. Stigmatization of and discrimination against obese individuals in the areas of employment, health care, and education have been demonstrated. Parental bias toward obese children has also been noted, and overweight adolescents are more likely to be socially isolated by their peers.[19] Recent data published by Yale University researchers show that even health care professionals who treat obese patients are biased against them and believe that these patients display stereotypical behaviors such as laziness that contribute to their weight gain.[20]

While weight gain causes health problems, weight loss has been shown to be beneficial. There are major health benefits when even 10 percent of body weight is lost and this weight loss is maintained. In fact, a landmark study conducted by the National Institutes of Health called the Diabetes Prevention Program (DPP) showed that a 5–7 percent weight loss through calorie restriction and moderate exercise in overweight subjects, with maintenance of this weight loss over three years, reduced the risk of progression to type 2 diabetes by 58 percent![21] These data show that you don't have to get back to what you weighed at the senior prom in order to derive significant medical benefit. In fact, unrealistic weight loss goals set us up for failure and are therefore counterproductive.

Because weight gain results in medical problems and weight loss can prevent the development of so many health problems, obesity should be considered a chronic medical condition, like high blood pressure or high cholesterol. Treatment of a chronic medical condition requires maintenance therapy to keep it under control. Just as blood pressure medications need to be continued to maintain the target blood pressure once it is achieved, so too lifestyle modification to maintain weight loss needs to be continued to keep your weight at goal. *Thus any weight loss intervention must be maintainable to be successful.* This point turns out to be critical, as you will see in Chapter 2 when fad diets are reviewed. If a diet can't be maintained over the long term, then it is useless, even if there is initial weight loss.

What's the best way to lose weight and keep it off? First you need to understand the process of weight gain. The human body tries to keep its net change in weight as close to zero as possible. However, even small imbalances due to increased caloric intake or decreased exercise can result in significant cumulative weight gain. In fact, it is estimated that the 20 pounds of weight the average American gains between the ages of twenty-five and fifty-five might be due to an imbalance as small as only 0.3 percent excess caloric intake.[22] To shed these pounds, therefore, you must reduce calories ingested and increase calories expended through exercise to tip the net caloric balance toward weight loss and then maintenance. The initial recommended weight loss goal should be about 10 percent of total body weight over approximately six months.[23] After the initial goal is met, further weight loss goals can then be established. For persons with a BMI between 27 and 35, a reduction of approximately 500 calories per day will result in the loss of one-half to one pound per week, leading to at least 10 percent cumulative weight loss in six months. For a BMI over 35, more calories will need to be trimmed (500–1,000 per day) to lose 10 percent body weight over six months simply because the absolute number of pounds representing 10 percent is higher.[24]

Ultimately, however, like all chronic medical conditions, prevention of obesity is easier and more effective than treatment. We must help our children avoid becoming overweight in the first place. It is important to recognize that calorie balance is precisely regulated by our bodies. Because small increases in calorie intake cause slow, gradual weight gain, minor healthy changes in eating habits and exercise can have a major impact on *preventing* weight gain. Based on the rate at which our population is gaining weight, it has been estimated that either reducing food intake by 100 calories per day or increasing calories burned through exercise by 100 per day could prevent the weight gain we are seeing in our society. This translates into walking an extra mile or taking a few less bites of food per day.[25]

Prevention is especially important for young people who are still at a healthy weight. Any intervention that encourages kids to eat less and exercise more should help. An easy target is television viewing and video game playing. Television likely results in an increased risk of obesity in children for several reasons. One is that kids who sit in front of the TV for hours each day are less physically active. Another is extra calories in the form of snacks eaten while watching TV. Kids may also be more likely to buy high-calorie foods and sugary soda as a result of the targeted TV advertising they are exposed to.[26] Whatever the reason, the number of hours of television watched by children has been shown to be directly correlated to an increased risk of obesity. The more time spent in front of the TV, the higher the risk of obesity. And it has been shown that reducing television time reduces the risk of weight gain.[27] This type of minor change in lifestyle needs to be championed by parents and school systems for prevention to become a reality. Personal example by parents and the right message from our public schools must be an integral part of instilling healthy diet and exercise habits in our children.

Government guidance regarding labeling and calorie intake is also critical. We probably have a lot to learn from the French in this regard. The French typically eat a diet high in fat and yet as a society historically have a lower incidence of obesity and heart disease than do other industrialized nations—a phenomenon called the French paradox. Many explanations have been proposed for this paradox, including the possible role of red wine. Although there are probably beneficial ingredients in wine, there are likely additional explanations. Perhaps smaller portions at meals—in stark contrast to our society of supersize portions, doggie bags, and the clean-plate club—are the key to the French paradox. As noted in a 2003 article in the *New York Times,* the French government supported programs in the early 1900s that promoted childhood dietary moderation. These programs may have prevented entire generations of French children from developing eating habits that would lead to obesity and heart disease. Simple measures such as set meal times supervised by adults, portion control, and restrictions on snacking may account at least in part for the mystery of the French paradox.[28] So in fact there is a track record for successful societal intervention to achieve the very minor lifestyle changes I have described to *prevent* weight gain. If you are concerned that these types of measures will take the pleasure out of eating, never fear. Observational studies have shown that although the French eat less than their American friends, they eat for longer periods of time.[29] In other words, they get more out of their food than we do. This may in part be due to eating meals in courses—another potential contributor to the French paradox. As you will see in Chapter 5, eating meals in courses is one practice we can emulate to try to reduce our calorie consumption.

For the moment, however, despite the availability of preventative measures that should be successful in preventing weight gain, there is little sign of anything other than continued worsening of the obesity epidemic. What will it take for us as a society to mobilize and foster healthy lifestyle changes that result in weight loss and therefore a reduction in the health risks associated with overweight and obesity? An article in the journal *Science* points out that political movements in the past have been able to catalyze social change only once a particular cause or issue was perceived as a crisis and a widespread threat to the public. In spite of recent media coverage of the health threats of obesity, this level of crisis is apparently not yet felt by the average citizen in this country.[30] Until the level of crisis that is indeed present is recognized, our society as a whole will likely sit back (with chips and dip in front of the television) and watch as a preventable epidemic burgeons.

The good news is that there is now some recognition of the weight gain crisis. A call to action for physicians who are on the front lines of the obesity epidemic was recently published in the *Archives of Internal Medicine,* with straightforward recommendations for diagnosis of overweight/obesity and counseling for weight loss. The hope is that a few minutes at each doctor visit will be spent helping patients lose weight. The authors recommend that information be given about exercise and basic dietary modification.[31] This is not always easy for the physician, who is frequently addressing multiple acute medical problems in the short period of time allotted to the patient visit and who therefore may forget or may not have time to discuss preventative health care issues such as weight loss. However, it is exactly a call to action of this type that has the potential to be a catalyst for change as just described. I can tell you that patients will not take a problem seriously if their physician does not. But if a problem such as overweight or obesity is given a higher profile during an office visit, the patient will recognize that this is a critical issue and not something to be ignored. A cartoon that ended a talk I recently attended portrayed a patient asking how much time he had left before he had to start paying attention to his doctor's recommendations. In the case of obesity, the answer is there is no time to waste.

As important as a call to action for physicians is, perhaps an even greater sign of a changing societal tide was an announcement by McDonald's on March 2, 2004, that the company would phase out the supersize french fry and soda options on their menus nationwide. I hope this will be only the start of a greater recognition that absurdly large portions should not be the norm, and that in spite of potential market-ing advantages, exploitation of the pervasive "more is better" mentality should not occur at the expense of our nation's health. I salute this deci-sion by the food industry to put our nation's health in front of profit.

This type of change can't come soon enough. Data from the Centers for Disease Control and Prevention (CDC) regarding causes of death in the United States in the year 2000 suggest that an estimated 400,000 preventable deaths resulted from poor diet and inactivity. This is up from 300,000 in 1990 and is significant not only because of the large absolute number of preventable deaths but also because the study's authors believe that these deaths will overtake smoking as the leading cause of preventable death in this country within the next few years "if the increasing trend of overweight is not reversed." Not only are the deaths theoretically preventable, but the trend would potentially be pre-ventable at the public health level through diet, exercise, and weight loss as a nation. Of interest is that smoking deaths were approximately unchanged from 1990.[32]

It is in the setting of this type of national mortality data and the recent class action lawsuits against tobacco companies that a lawsuit has been brought (and at this point thrown out) against the fast-food indus-try seeking damages for the alleged role the industry plays in causing teenage weight gain. On March 10, 2004, the United States House of Representatives approved the Personal Responsibility in Food Con-sumption Act. This legislation holds the consumer responsible for his or her own weight gain and prevents lawsuits from being brought by con-sumers blaming their weight gain on the food industry. At the time this book went to press the bill has not yet been voted on by the United States Senate. Proponents of this legislation believe the individual is responsible for what he or she eats and that this legislation will prevent frivolous class action lawsuits. Opponents feel that the bill sends a mes-sage to the food industry that it does not need to concern itself with pub-lic health issues.[33] Whatever the fate of this legislation, it is clear that weight gain in the United States is starting to get noticed on the national political stage. Hopefully as a result of such debate, positive changes in people's eating behaviors and positive changes in the food industry such as the supersize phase-out will follow.

Perhaps the day when Americans will recognize the level of crisis the obesity epidemic represents is drawing closer. We can only hope that the health risks of overweight and obesity eventually get the same attention that smoking, drunk driving, seat belts, and bicycle helmets have received in the recent past. Maybe over the next months and years we will become a more health-focused nation, with action against weight gain starting to take center stage.

THE SOCIOECONOMICS OF OVERWEIGHT AND OBESITY

While the rest of this book is directed toward helping *you* lose weight, I want to briefly address the current socioeconomics of obesity.

A special article in the January 2004 issue of the *American Journal of Clinical Nutrition* points out that the highest rates of obesity occur among the poor and least educated in our country. The authors note that this is in no small part due to the fact that energy-dense foods are obtainable at a lower cost to the consumer than healthier food choices.[34] Right now in this country it is less expensive to eat unhealthy, calorie-dense foods that cause weight gain. Until this bottom line changes, we will likely be fighting a losing battle. The basic theory of supply and demand tells us that the more a good or service (healthy fresh food) costs, the less people consume, whereas the cheaper a good or service (less nutritious and more calorie-dense food) is, the more they consume. Another applicable economic principle in this respect is that of inferior goods. There are certain products, termed inferior goods, that consumers buy less of as their income increases. Conversely, consumers buy more of these so-called inferior goods as their income decreases. Ironically and unfortunately, the classic example given for an inferior good is calorie-dense cheap food.

Thus we are up against powerful economic forces. Even with all the data in the world supporting the benefits of a healthy diet, we may very well make no headway in our battle against weight gain until we address the eating patterns of poverty, both because the economically disadvantaged are less likely to have the luxury of being concerned with delayed health benefits when more immediate concerns such as the day-to-day costs of living take precedence and because of phenomena such as the purchasing of inferior goods. We, as a nation, need to make fresh, healthy foods available at a lower cost to all consumers. In the long run it will cost our society less than paying to treat the health consequences of overweight and obesity.

The American way is to provide what the market demands. We as consumers, therefore, need to create a demand for inexpensive healthy food. The rest of the solution must be addressed by the federal government (including the Department of Agriculture) and the food industry. Let us insist on providing our nation with food of *superior* quality so that our economically disadvantaged citizens don't resort to consuming inferior goods.

Chapter 2

WHY FAD DIETS DON'T WORK

*I*nstantaneous solutions, although enticing, never solve problems. Get-rich-quick schemes don't fool us; why should lose-weight-quick schemes be any different? If it sounds too good to be true, it is. Don't let impatience and unrealistic expectations derail your best efforts. Look around at the successful tennis player, the successful violinist, and the successful businessperson. They got where they are through hard work, lots of it, and it wasn't always pleasant. Any one of them will say that there were more than minor sacrifices along the way. I'm not telling you anything you don't already know. Why, then, do we all expect weight loss to be any different? We need to realize that it will not be instantaneous, it will not always be easy, and it will require some sacrifices along the way. I can tell you that no other person or product is going to lose weight for you. What you should know, however, is that weight loss is quite possible with the right game plan. In fact, a good game plan is the critical piece that is usually missing in failed attempts to lose weight, and that's what I provide for you in this book.

Popular or "fad" diets in various forms and flavors have

existed for decades, each diet claiming that it has the unique formula to solve our nation's weight problem. I argue that the very fact that these diets have been present while the obesity epidemic has exploded in this country is in itself evidence that they are not the answer to the problem.

Regardless of whether strict adherence to a dietary formula results in weight loss, if a person is unable to maintain compliance with the diet, then it is ultimately a failure. This has been shown to be the case with popular diets that require dramatic alteration in calorie intake or in the types and/or quality of food eaten; these are simply not maintainable beyond several months. Once a person is unable for any reason to maintain the recommended dietary changes, the weight lost is quickly regained.

Recently published data have shown that although there may be significant weight loss with fad diets such as low-carbohydrate diets, the weight loss is transient. And though there may be cardiovascular benefit associated with the weight loss on these diets, these benefits are limited to the time a patient can maintain the diet and are lost thereafter. For example, a recent study showed that any weight loss advantage at six months associated with a low-carbohydrate diet was lost at one year.[1] Additionally, calorie intake, not the nutrient composition of any diet, is the major determinant of weight loss.[2] A recent review of the published medical literature on low-carbohydrate diets concluded that not only is there insufficient evidence to recommend low-carb diets but the weight lost on such diets was due to the resultant calorie restriction and not to the reduced carbohydrate content.[3] This finding is in keeping with a small study of forty-three obese patients back in 1996. In that study all patients consumed 1,000 calories per day, but the carbohydrate composition of the patients' diets varied from 15 to 45 percent of total daily calories. There was no difference in the amount of weight lost (about 17½ pounds in six weeks) regardless of the percentage of daily calories from carbs.[4] In other words, it's calorie restriction, not carbohydrate restriction in and of itself, that results in weight loss.

Not only does widely publicized data continue to emerge supporting no long-term weight loss advantage to low-carbohydrate diets,[5] but not all the weight initially lost on fad diets is fat. Diets very high in protein and fat and low in carbohydrates result in more body water loss than body fat loss in the short term, resulting in the typically deceiving dramatic weight loss at their onset. Additionally, dramatic carbohydrate restriction is counter to the advice of government agencies such as the

United States Department of Agriculture (USDA) and the National Institutes of Health (NIH). Very low carbohydrate diets are nutritionally inadequate and are lacking in dietary fiber, folate, calcium, magnesium, potassium, and vitamins A, E, and B$_1$.[6] Another concern that has been largely overlooked by the public is the effect such diets have on calcium metabolism. There is data suggesting that the increased acid load that high-protein diets deliver to the body causes an abnormality in calcium excretion at the kidney. This results in negative calcium balance and possibly an increased risk of kidney stones and bone loss.[7] Thus people with previous kidney stones or significant osteoporosis may be unnecessarily putting themselves at further risk with diets that are high in protein and very low in carbohydrates. High levels of meat and seafood consumption have also been shown to increase the risk of gout.[8]

What about the mood swings and fatigue we hear people blaming on carbohydrate consumption? Interestingly, Massachusetts Institute of Technology (MIT) researchers and others have found that low-carbohydrate diets adversely affect serotonin levels in the brain, resulting in irritability. This effect on brain serotonin levels also results in diminished satiety (feeling full after meals).[9]

I address the specifics of carbohydrates and weight loss in Chapter 4, but for the moment I want to talk a little more about carbohydrates in general and for that matter meats. Maybe I'm alone here, but it just seems ridiculous to recommend elimination (or close to it) of all carbohydrates in our diet. It seems equally silly to recommend eliminating all meat from our diet. Let's think about this for a moment. The domestication of wheat and the development of farming may have been the historical event that allowed civilization as we know it to develop. Wheat has been around for a long time, far longer than the epidemic of overweight and obesity that we are witnessing. Additionally, historically the cultures with some of the lowest heart disease rates in the world ate meat. The members of hunter-gatherer cultures such as the !Kung (the "!"signifies a clicking sound) got plenty of exercise, ate diets with carbohydrates that were high in fiber, and ate wild game that had not undergone selective breeding (as has our domesticated meat) for meat high in fat content. So although they ate meat and carbohydrates, it was of a very different variety than we are used to today. When the !Kung moved to cities and adopted the local diet and a sedentary lifestyle, they began to develop heart disease because, as noted in our first chapter, they were thrown into an environment they were not suited for (as were we all).

The obesity epidemic is relatively new. So things such as carbohydrates and meat in general aren't the sole culprits here. It's the type and quantity of these foods against the backdrop of a sedentary lifestyle that is responsible. In other words, it's just too easy to blame and eliminate a certain food group. This is not addressing the problem, and as you will see below, eliminating entire food groups from your diet is not maintainable in any event, so it isn't an option even if it were appropriate. Let's make an analogy. Antibiotics aren't responsible for the outbreak of antibiotic resistance we now see in bacteria. It's their overuse and misuse that has caused the problem. Our reaction isn't (and for that matter shouldn't be) "don't use antibiotics." Our reaction is and should be to use antibiotics responsibly so that we can prevent further problems. Use antibiotics when appropriate and you will save lives. So let's not blame wheat, carbohydrates, and meat for our problems. Let's eat them responsibly and balance our diets with carbohydrates high in fiber and lean meats that have been shown to be healthy for us.

An entire issue of the *American Journal of Clinical Nutrition* in the fall of 2003 was dedicated to studies showing that whole grains actually decrease the development of diabetes and heart disease. That is, it's OK to eat carbohydrates. So if you want to blame wheat, blame its domestication, which resulted in our modern civilization with technologies that allow us to live sedentary lifestyles, but don't blame carbs in and of themselves. I do agree that processed carbohydrates and sugars are not good choices. Briefly, in addition to their high calorie density, these processed carbohydrates have a high glycemic index that *may* also contribute to medical problems and difficulty with weight loss. I will address why some carbohydrates are better than others in Chapter 4. But let's get back to fad diets in general for the moment.

Of great interest is a presentation at the American Heart Association meeting in November 2003 by Tufts University researchers describing a study of 160 patients on four different diets (Weight Watchers, Atkins, Ornish, and the Zone). While patients were on these respective diets, they lost weight and reduced their risk of heart disease. However, the diets were not maintainable. As an example, up to 50 percent of patients on the Atkins diet and the Ornish diet dropped out.[10] The results from this study reemphasize my message that although different diets may be helpful when followed carefully, they are essentially useless unless they are maintainable. Fad or popular diets fail this test.

In 2001 the United States Department of Agriculture published a comprehensive review of fad diets and concluded that traditional low-calorie diets were best for sustained weight loss.[11] This seems obvious, but in spite of this dieters continue to try to lose weight with fad diets. They keep trying new fad diets because of a desire to lose weight quickly and easily. Additionally, dieters select a goal weight for appearance and sense of physical comfort rather than health considerations or medical reasons and thus tend to try diets that promise quick and dramatic weight loss.[12] People also have a tendency to believe weight loss philosophies that are not supported by our understanding of human physiology and are not backed by any scientific literature. They are frequently taken in by the promise of quick initial weight loss only to be disappointed when the fad diet is not maintainable and weight is regained. The human body will fight to maintain its established weight set point, and this makes quick weight loss doomed to failure.

It is not surprising, therefore, that researchers have noted that high day-to-day fluctuation in food intake and rigid control of eating habits are paradoxically counterproductive and disrupt more appropriate food choice behaviors.[13] This makes sustainable weight loss more difficult. Lifestyle changes that allow for individuals to concentrate on their daily routine are a more effective approach to weight loss. The recurrent scenario I see in the clinic every day is that the patients who lose weight and keep it off are those who go for a modest alteration in calories, eat high-quality foods (high-fiber carbohydrates, healthy meats, and unsaturated fats), and establish and keep up with an exercise program. Because modest adjustments in diet are maintainable, the weight loss that results is also maintainable.

It is telling that the word *diet* derives from the Greek *diaita,* meaning "manner of living." It is a change in manner of living or lifestyle that is necessary to lose weight and maintain weight loss. This book's premise is that this change in manner of living involves not just a change in eating habits but a change in *overeating* habits—a distinction that on the surface may sound trivial but is in fact critical. Calories that are derived from overeating are a large contributor to the total daily calorie count and can be cut carefully without causing significant hunger. Cutting these extra calories is covered in depth in upcoming chapters and is the cornerstone of our dietary recommendations. By making several minor changes in your approach to overeating, the necessary calorie reduction to achieve gradual and consistent weight loss that is maintainable will be well within your reach.

The National Weight Control Registry, established by nationally renowned obesity researchers, is a collection of thousands of individuals who have been successful in significant weight loss and maintenance.[14] This registry collects data to determine what dietary and exercise habits people who lose weight have in common, and it should therefore give insight into what lends itself to a successful weight loss program. Individuals were enrolled if they had lost 30 pounds or more and had maintained this loss for at least one year.[15] Several interesting findings have emerged from this database. These registry participants are eating fewer calories and fewer calories from fat than people in the general U.S. population.[16] People in the registry who regained weight reported an increase in fat intake and less exercise.[17] Participants also report that weight loss improves self-confidence and physical and psychological well-being.[18]

You may say, "Tell me something that I don't know." My point here is that there is evidence showing that fad dieters can't maintain their weight loss because of an inability to stick to their diet, but that basic and moderate lifestyle modification *is* maintainable and results in long-term, successful weight loss. In fact, the National Weight Control Registry members in one report had lost an average of 66 pounds and maintained this loss over five years.[19] Additionally, the registry reveals that the longer weight is kept off, the easier it becomes to keep it off.[20] Thus there is good science backing up what happens to also be common sense. So let's put what we claim to already know into practice.

Our purpose in writing *The Nantucket Diet* is to provide the estimated 65 percent of overweight or obese adult Americans with an alternative dietary strategy for weight loss and maintenance. Specifically, it is an alternative to the numerous popular fad diets that feed off the American quick-fix psyche and result in quick but unsustainable weight loss. *The Nantucket Diet* is a product of the scientific literature and everyday life experience. The Nantucket Diet plan makes physiologic sense, is maintainable beyond the three-to-six-month period after which fad dieters typically burn out, and is in line with evidence published in peer-reviewed medical journals and with national obesity guidelines published by the NIH. Our emphasis will be on lifestyle modification surrounding overeating, food choices, and exercise. I have seen patients who follow the recommendations in this book meet with long-term success, and am confident you will join their ranks.

Chapter 3

DOES THE TYPE OF FOOD MATTER?
YES!

$\mathscr{A}$utopsies done on young American soldiers who lost their lives fighting in the Korean and Vietnam Wars revealed that between 45 and 77 percent had coronary artery disease at the time of their death. Six percent of these young soldiers already had what was considered to be severe coronary artery disease at autopsy. Another autopsy study of young Americans reported in 1993 revealed the same approximate percentages of heart disease.[1] These data tell us that the heart disease process starts at a very young age in our country and progresses over our lifetimes. It is not surprising, therefore, that heart disease is our country's number one killer.

How have we moved from our hunting and gathering origins to a society where heart disease is already taking hold in childhood? Most now believe this phenomenon is due to relatively recent dietary changes and a sedentary lifestyle—the same dietary changes and sedentary lifestyle that did in fact result in the development of heart disease even in the !Kung as they were assimilated into industrialized society. What specific changes in our diets are responsible for the development of heart disease remains a matter of debate, although it shouldn't, because the facts are clear: diets high in calories and certain fats and low in fiber lead to coronary disease. This occurs through many mechanisms, one of which is a resultant elevation in cholesterol. Is fat consumption the sole culprit? Is all fat bad for you? The discussion as to how much and which fats are bad for you clearly did not end with the highly publicized debates in the 1970s and 1980s between Dr. Pritikin (an advocate of a low-fat diet) and Dr. Atkins (who recommended replacing carbohydrates with fat and protein). In fact, if anything, the debate is the fiercest it has ever been.

If one reviews the scientific literature regarding which type of popular diet plan is best for the heart, it is often noted that there are not many large or long-term studies in this regard. I beg to differ. What about a study looking at the history of modern humankind? Here is how the abstract might appear in a modern medical journal:

Heart Healthy Diet: A Retrospective Cohort
Mother Nature et al.

BACKGROUND: Modern humans have been around for a long time. Their bodies are designed to eat certain types of foods.

METHODS: Mother Nature has recruited all of humankind for hundreds of thousands of years and given them high-fiber carbohydrates, lean meats, and fish combined with ample exercise.

RESULTS: Coronary heart disease is essentially nonexistent in traditional hunter-gatherer societies.

CONCLUSIONS: Foods that we have been eating for hundreds of thousands of years combined with exercise prevent heart disease. There is nothing we can do to change that.

In other words, a diet of high-fiber carbohydrates, lean meat, and fish, combined with exercise, has been clearly shown to prevent heart disease throughout our evolutionary history. So before we lose perspective arguing about which fad diet is best for the heart, let's remember that over 50,000 years of experience ain't no fad. I'm not suggesting that we all go back to live in the forest and get rid of our cars (although that might be a good thing for the environment). That was then and this is now. I am, however, suggesting that there is no replacement for healthy carbohydrates, lean meats, and exercise if we intend to prevent heart disease. So the next time you hear someone arguing about data for a particular fad diet lowering heart disease risk, remind that person about the largest and longest study ever conducted.

This chapter presents a general guide to healthy eating. What is critical to understand is that the types and amounts of food you eat will have a dramatic effect on your health, both indirectly through weight gain and directly through effects on a wide range of illnesses such as heart disease and cancer. Data from the scientific literature supports the notion that while you are progressing through the three phases of the Nantucket Diet it is important not just to reduce calories but to pay attention to the types and quality of food you are eating. This issue is complex, but there is compelling evidence that you should avoid foods high in saturated and trans fats and eat carbohydrates high in fiber. Long-term population data across several Western countries show that the consumption of foods derived from animal sources such as butter, meat, and lard is associated with an increased risk of death from heart disease, whereas the consumption of vegetables and fish is associated with a lower risk of death from heart disease.[2] Likewise, increased consumption of vegetables and consumption of less fat from animal sources in rural China has been associated with a dramatically decreased risk of heart disease when compared to the typical high-fat, low-fiber American diet,[3] and a recently published study from India found that increased vegetable consumption protects against heart disease.[4]

Fats can cause trouble in two ways. Compared to protein and carbohydrates, fat has the highest number of calories per gram and therefore the highest calorie density. So independent of any effect specific fats might have on heart health, fats in general can easily lead to weight gain and the resultant insulin resistance we will discuss in Chapter 4. Saturated and trans fats have also been shown to raise the level of LDL (bad) cholesterol. High LDL cholesterol has been clearly shown to be a risk factor for heart disease, and lowering LDL cholesterol has been shown in many large clinical trials to lower the risk of heart disease. It makes sense, then, that reduced fat consumption, likely through its effect on cholesterol and other factors, has been shown to lower heart disease risk.[5] So high fat intake in general is a risk factor for obesity and heart disease, certain types of fats can raise your cholesterol, and decreasing fat consumption can lower your heart disease risk. Conversely, with respect to carbohydrates, there is evidence that diets high in whole-grain carbohydrates and fiber reduce the risk of heart disease.[6] What isn't

100 percent clear, however, is the exact components of whole grain that provide this benefit, and the mechanism of this effect still remains a matter to be established.

Thus there still remains controversy as to what the primary contributor to weight gain and heart disease is—bad fats or refined carbohydrates. The truth is that it's probably a combination of the two. The bottom line, therefore, is that the evidence suggests that both reduction in saturated and trans fats and increasing whole grains and fiber will help prevent weight gain and heart disease.

So what should you eat and how much of it? The recommendations can vary slightly depending on whom you ask. Even the lingo has changed. The old RDAs (Recommended Daily Allowances) that we remember from childhood have been replaced by DRIs (Dietary Reference Intakes). This new terminology was reiterated by the Institute of Medicine in 2002[7] and moves us from maximum consumption per day to accepted ranges.[8] It is suggested that adults get 45–65 percent of their daily calories from carbohydrates, 10–35 percent from protein, and 20–35 percent from fat. Other organizations such as the American Heart Association have guidelines that are similar. What I think is more important than exact percentages is the approximate percentage of each food group and the types of food eaten. With this in mind, the following recommendations apply:

- **Eat carbohydrates high in fiber.** Fiber is plant material that we can't digest. Foods high in fiber include vegetables, fruits, beans, and whole-grain breads and cereals. Whole-grain products are made from all three components of the grain kernel: the outer covering, or bran; the middle layer, or germ; and the inner portion, or endosperm. Refined flour in products such as white bread may have a softer texture but is made only from the endosperm, losing the valuable fiber and nutrients from the germ and bran layers.

  There are two different types of fiber, each with its own health benefits. Insoluble fiber found in foods such as cabbage, beets, carrots, whole wheat, and wheat bran helps with constipation and may reduce the risk of colon cancer. Soluble fiber found in foods such as oats, beans, peas, apples, and strawberries helps lower cholesterol and may improve blood sugar levels.

Many fruits, vegetables, and beans contain both types of fiber, and as just mentioned, high fiber intake in general has been associated with a decreased risk of heart disease. The American Heart Association (AHA) recommends five servings of fruit and vegetables per day (count avocado and olives as fats), with a goal of 25–30 grams of fiber per day.[9] Choose oats, barley, and whole-grain breads and pasta.

- **Try to limit fat intake in general and saturated and trans fats specifically. Choose foods high in monounsaturated and poly-unsaturated fats.** As a general rule, saturated fats are solid at room temperature (with the exception of some tropical oils, such as coconut and palm kernel oil), and mono- and polyunsaturated fats are liquid or soft at room temperature. Try to avoid butter and lard as well as oils high in saturated fats such as coconut oil, as they can raise cholesterol. I recommend olive or canola oil. Avoid trans fatty acids, found in partially hydrogenated oils, as they can raise cholesterol. These fats occur in most vegetable shortening and in fried or baked prepackaged and processed foods. I recommend avoiding most stick margarines. Avoid dairy products that are not reduced-fat. Consider lean meats that are low in total fat and saturated fat, such as lean beef, turkey, skinless chicken, wild game, bison, and ostrich.[10] The American Heart Association recommends that saturated plus trans fats should not be more than 10 percent of total daily calories. For processed or packaged foods you can use information on food labels to determine the number of calories from the different types of fats. Thus if you are eating 1,500 calories per day, you don't want to eat more than 150 calories from saturated fats and trans fats in one day. This leaves the rest of the daily total of 30 percent fat from mono- and polyunsaturated fats. Almonds, peanuts, pecans, and walnuts are good sources of monounsaturated fats; they also are good sources of protein and other nutrients. Remember, however, that fats in general, including those in nuts, have a high calorie density, and therefore healthy fats should replace calories from unhealthy foods. I am not saying that you should never eat meat or butter again—I'm just recommending that you eat them in moderation.

Fish, particularly fatty fish, is good for your heart. Eat at least two servings of fatty fish, rich in omega-3 oils, each week, as discussed in more detail at the end of this chapter.

Do the recommendations just noted prevent heart disease in the real world? The answer is yes. A recent scientific review of the medical literature studying the relationship between diet and heart disease revealed that there are certain dietary patterns that are associated with a lower risk of heart disease. This study found that diets featuring predominantly unsaturated fats, carbohydrates that are primarily from whole grains, lots of vegetables and fruit, and omega-3 fatty acids protected against heart disease.[11] The traditional diets of the Mediterranean region, including Greece and Italy (whole-grain cereals, vegetables, fruit, nuts, legumes, and moderate amounts of fish as well as significant olive oil intake, low saturated-fat intake, low to moderate dairy consumption, and wine with meals), include the types of foods found to be heart-protective in the above-noted review. In fact, a large study looking at the dietary habits of over twenty-five thousand Europeans found that the more closely people adhered to the traditional Mediterranean diet, the lower their risk of death due to heart disease (reduced by 33 percent) and death due to cancer (reduced by 26 percent).[12] So there is evidence that these traditional Mediterranean dietary patterns result in a lower risk of death from heart disease, and many health care professionals therefore recommend the above types of foods to their patients. I believe these foods should be incorporated into any diet. Although theoretically all that matters for weight loss is calorie reduction, there is evidence that the type of food matters as well for disease prevention. The great thing is that the same foods that are good for you also fit nicely into our weight loss program. Foods high in fiber happen to also be low in calorie density and therefore make weight loss easier.

A traditional Mediterranean dietary scheme is well represented in the food pyramid shown on the next page.

This type of specialized food pyramid is of great interest, as there has been significant controversy recently regarding the validity of what many view as the now obsolete USDA food pyramid. Issues raised include the alleged failure of the USDA pyramid to recognize that not all fats are bad for you and that not all carbohydrates are good for you. Researchers at Harvard Medical School have proposed a revised pyramid with less emphasis on refined carbohydrates and more emphasis on

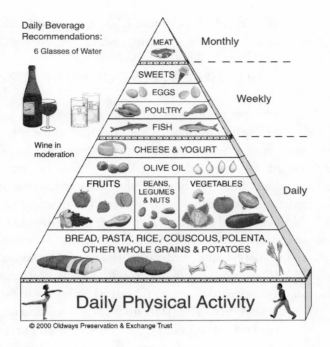

Daily Beverage Recommendations:
6 Glasses of Water

MEAT — Monthly

SWEETS

EGGS

POULTRY — Weekly

FISH

Wine in moderation

CHEESE & YOGURT

OLIVE OIL

FRUITS | BEANS, LEGUMES & NUTS | VEGETABLES — Daily

BREAD, PASTA, RICE, COUSCOUS, POLENTA, OTHER WHOLE GRAINS & POTATOES

Daily Physical Activity

© 2000 Oldways Preservation & Exchange Trust

whole-grain foods, and mono- and polyunsaturated fats.[13] Should these changes be implemented, the new USDA pyramid might look a lot more like the Mediterranean pyramid shown above. The USDA has in fact decided to reevaluate its food pyramid and has addressed this potential revision in several recent meetings.[14] In the meantime, in addition to the Mediterranean pyramid there are several other specialty pyramids that allow for variation in food choices and address social and cultural preferences. These pyramids (vegetarian, Asian) can be found at the Web site of the nonprofit group Oldways at www.oldwayspt.org.

In summary, there are to this point only claims, unsubstantiated by large studies, that fad diets that replace almost all carbohydrates with bacon, meat, butter, and other foods high in saturated fats prevent heart disease. To the contrary, there is data suggesting that these same saturated fats lead to heart disease. In addition, in contrast to fad diets that recommend eliminating almost all carbohydrates, there is data that whole grains and other carbohydrates high in fiber, such as vegetables, are associated with decreased heart disease risk. So not only are there compelling data from large studies that diets that include healthy fats and carbohydrates can prevent heart disease and cancer, but these foods fit perfectly into a weight loss program given their low calorie density. These are the types of food we recommend.

ALCOHOL: HEALTH BUZZ OR JUST A BUZZ?

What about drinking alcohol as a means of preventing heart disease? There has certainly been a lot of recent attention in the media about the possible benefits of moderate drinking. The answer is probably not as straightforward as you think. How alcohol may be heart-protective, which type of alcohol may be best, the amount needed to derive the putative benefit, or whether there is in fact a clear benefit are all controversial.[15] Although drinking alcohol in moderation may lower heart disease risk in certain persons, the lack of definitive data and the risk of alcoholism and its resultant medical costs and social ramifications have led the AHA to recommend that *current* drinkers consume alcohol in moderation, not more than one to two drinks per day for men and one drink per day for women. The AHA goes on to recommend that people who do not already drink should not start drinking to prevent heart disease.[16] I recommend no more than one drink per day for men or women who currently drink and agree that nondrinkers should not start drinking alcohol to protect their hearts. Let's also not forget that alcohol can contain a significant number of calories!

SUPPLEMENTS: ARE YOU GETTING YOUR MONEY'S WORTH?

There are many dietary supplements that are now available on the U.S. market, some with better evidence for beneficial health effects than others. The putative benefits of these dietary supplements range from heart health to cancer prevention. I will only address two of these supplements in depth in this chapter, antioxidants and fish oil. Both have been evaluated in well-designed scientific studies. The former has not been shown to have any clear benefit, and the latter appears to have a clear beneficial effect on heart health.

Antioxidants have received a lot of enthusiastic endorsement by their manufacturers for their alleged benefit in preventing heart disease and cancer. Although there are certainly theories that can be brought forth as possible mechanisms of action for this type of heart protection, at this point the American Heart Association's position is that there is not good enough evidence to recommend antioxidant supplements for the prevention of disease.[17] The alleged preventative properties of antioxidant supplements have been studied in large clinical trials. Vitamin E at 400 units per day over four and a half years was found to have no heart-protective effect in patients at high risk for heart disease, including patients with diabetes.[18] An additional study looking at over twenty thousand patients with heart disease or diabetes who took 600 mg of vitamin E, 250 mg of vitamin C, and 20 mg of beta-carotene daily for five years revealed no reduction in heart disease, stroke, or cancer risk.[19] Thus at this time the data suggest that antioxidant vitamins at the doses and duration taken in the above studies provide no heart disease or cancer protection.

As it turns out, however, an individual's genetic makeup may determine whether antioxidants prevent disease. Recent data out of the Technion Institute in Israel suggest that variations in a blood protein called haptoglobin may help identify which individuals taking antioxidants will receive a beneficial effect. This is the type of data that may one day be available to doctors to help them select patients who will benefit from specific drugs. Thus the answer may in fact be that antioxidants will have benefit in some people and not others.[20]

What about fish oil supplements? Beneficial omega-3 fatty acids are found in oily fish such as tuna, salmon, sardines, mackerel, and bluefish. The omega-3 fatty acids eicosapentaenoic acid (EPA) and docosahexaenoic acid (DHA) found in these fish have been shown to prevent death from heart disease.[21] These fish oils may exert their effect through a direct beneficial effect on the heart and blood vessels or through beneficial effects on blood platelets and cholesterol.[22] Whatever the mechanism, these fish oils are in fact recommended by the American Heart Association for the prevention of heart disease. The AHA recommends at least two servings of fatty fish per week for healthy adults (pregnant women or women considering pregnancy or breast-feeding should consult their doctor before eating these fish). Patients with established heart disease or certain types of high cholesterol should discuss fish oil supplements with their doctors.[23]

I suggest healthy people try to get their omega-3 through diet, i.e., the types of fish noted above. If you wish to take supplements because you dislike fish or have a strong family history of heart disease, discuss omega-3 supplementation with your physician.

What about over-the-counter dietary supplements marketed for weight loss? A recent extensive review of the topic looked at several over-the-counter dietary supplements, including chitosan, chromium picolinate, guar gum, and hydroxy-methylbutyrate. Ironically, the only dietary supplement found to have data "beyond a reasonable doubt" suggesting help with weight loss was ephedra, which was banned by the Food and Drug Administration at the end of 2003 because of its connection to adverse health events.[24]

The take-home message from this chapter is that your food choices have an impact on your weight and your health. I have described the types of foods that are not only *healthy* but are also *helpful* for weight loss. We have followed this philosophy when choosing the recipes for our book. They are both healthy and delicious—examples of good food that can be good for you!

Chapter 4

INSULIN, CARBOHYDRATES, AND DIABETES

*N*ews flash: insulin is a good thing. Insulin, a hormone made in the pancreas that regulates blood sugar, is not only life-sustaining for type 1 (previously called juvenile) diabetics but is an indispensable tool for treating high blood sugar in type 2 diabetics. Insulin is far more potent than any of the oral diabetic medications, and tight blood sugar control with insulin treatment has been shown to prevent or delay damage to diabetics' eyes, kidneys, and feet. In addition, aggressive insulin therapy in the hospital has been shown to decrease the risk of death in patients who have had heart attacks and in patients who have been admitted to the intensive care unit.[1] It is resistance to or decreased response to insulin in our fat tissue, muscle, and liver that causes problems. This phenomenon is called insulin resistance.

Insulin resistance occurs as the result of weight gain. As we gain weight, particularly in the abdominal area, our bodies' metabolism changes and the insulin we produce doesn't work as well as it should. A normal pancreas increases its insulin production to try to overcome this insulin resistance and keep the body's blood sugar levels normal. This results in high insulin levels in the blood. *Therefore a high insulin level in the blood is not the original cause of obesity, but itself is a result of obesity and is a marker of the insulin resistance syndrome.* Although it is true that insulin treatment can cause weight gain and insulin has many different actions in our tissues at the cellular level, suggesting that a high blood insulin level per se is the devil that causes our weight gain problems is backward thinking. What *is* the case is that weight loss will improve insulin resistance and as a result will lower insulin levels because the pancreas needs to produce less insulin in response to meals and on awakening to keep blood sugar levels normal.

Insulin resistance is in fact the core problem in obesity and is felt to be the cause of the increased risk of heart disease and stroke that results. The group of metabolic abnormalities associated with obesity that lead to heart disease have been given several names, including insulin resistance syndrome, dysmetabolic syndrome, metabolic syndrome, and syndrome X. The insulin resistance syndrome causes heart disease indirectly through its unhealthy effects on cholesterol levels, blood pressure, and blood clotting as well as directly through its interference with normal artery wall function. These problems surface—and the risk of heart disease rises—long before the pancreas starts to fail and a patient develops diabetes. Doctors should now know that it is critical to recognize the insulin resistance syndrome even before their patients develop diabetes. In fact, the National Cholesterol Education Program's Adult Treatment Panel has developed guidelines to diagnose the insulin resistance syndrome. A patient has to have only three of the risk factors listed on the next page to qualify for the insulin resistance syndrome.

It is critical for doctors and other health care professionals to make this risk assessment early because it has been shown that a patient who meets the above criteria for the insulin resistance syndrome has at least double the risk of dying from heart disease.[2] Once insulin resistance is identified, diet, exercise, weight loss, and treatment of cholesterol and blood pressure are critical to prevent heart attack or stroke.

As part of the movement to identify individuals with the insulin resistance syndrome earlier, a person who has a fasting blood sugar of over 99 is now diagnosed with prediabetes.[3] Estimates from the U.S. Department of Health and Human Services put the number of Americans with prediabetes at over forty million. Prediabetes is a sign of insulin resistance and is also associated with a high risk of progression

DIAGNOSING THE INSULIN RESISTANCE SYNDROME

Risk Factor	Defining Level
• Abdominal obesity (waist circumference)	
Men	>102 cm (>40 in)
Women	>88 cm (>35 in)
• Triglycerides	≥150 mg/dL
• High-density lipoprotein cholesterol (HDL)	
Men	<40 mg/dL
Women	<50 mg/dL
• Blood pressure	≥130/≥86 mm Hg
• Fasting glucose	≥110 mg/dL

Source: NHLBI, Executive Summary, NCEP ATP III; JAMA, May 16, 2001; 285(19): 2486.

to diabetes. This is a critical distinction not only for treatment of choles-terol and blood pressure to prevent heart attack but because a large National Institutes of Health study showed that a 5–7 percent weight loss through diet and moderate exercise can reduce by 58 percent the risk of progression to diabetes.[4] I'll take this opportunity to note that there is no such thing as "borderline diabetes." If your fasting blood sugar is over 125 mg/dl on two occasions, diabetes is diagnosed. Any attempt to use euphemisms such as "a touch of the sugar" or "border-line diabetes" to describe an elevated blood sugar is simply ignoring the currently accepted criteria for the diagnosis of type 2 diabetes.

As we gain weight our bodies become more insulin-resistant. The body's resultant high insulin levels are a marker of this insulin resistance syndrome and its associated increased risk of heart disease and stroke. Diets that propose to "balance" insulin levels by dramatically restricting carbohydrates are not directly affecting insulin resistance; they are sim-ply providing less stimulus for the pancreas to produce insulin. The real sign of progress is when a carbohydrate load elicits less insulin secretion as a result of previous weight loss; this is an indication that a patient's insulin resistance has improved. Thus instead of avoiding stress to a bro-ken system by lowering carbohydrate intake, the answer is to fix the system by losing weight so it responds properly to stress. A body that doesn't need to produce large amounts of insulin to keep blood sugar levels normal is a body that is less insulin-resistant and therefore less likely to have the associated cholesterol, blood pressure, and arterial wall function abnormalities. A body that has all the insulin resistance problems mentioned above will continue to be at risk for heart disease regardless of whether lower insulin levels are achieved with carbohydrate restriction. As you read in the first chapter, low-carbohydrate diets seem to cause weight loss because of their resultant calorie restriction. So as with any weight loss, insulin resistance will improve, but not as a direct result of the carbohydrate restriction. If, as I've reviewed in Chapter 2, an individual cannot maintain the dramatic lifestyle changes required by fad diets, including low-carbohydrate diets, weight regain will occur, and with it insulin resistance will again worsen.

So what about all the hype demonizing carbohydrates and suggesting that they cause weight gain through their effect on insulin stimulation? As I have just discussed, high insulin levels are themselves the result of obesity and the resulting insulin resistance, not the cause. There is data suggesting that not all carbohydrates are created equal. A measure called the glycemic index predicts how much effect a particular carbohydrate will have on your blood sugar (and as a result how much insulin is secreted by the pancreas in response). As a general rule, the higher the fiber content of a carbohydrate, the lower its glycemic index. For example, whole grains have a low glycemic index. Bread made with refined white flour will have a higher glycemic index. The higher a food's glycemic index, the higher the insulin response to that food. A study of overweight teenage boys in Boston showed that meals with a high glycemic load (glycemic load takes the glycemic index and *amount* of carbohydrate into consideration) resulted in higher insulin levels and perhaps relatively lower blood sugar levels after meals. This drop in blood sugar may have resulted in hunger and therefore indirectly resulted in an increased calorie intake after meals, resulting in further weight gain. Because of this cascade of events, the authors of this study hypothesized that attempts at weight loss would be more difficult for people who eat lots of refined carbohydrates.[5]

Eating a lot of carbohydrates with a high glycemic index may in fact make it harder to lose weight via this mechanism, but this has yet to be determined definitively. What doesn't change, however, is that weight loss must be achieved through calorie reduction. The weight gain hypothesized to occur with high-glycemic-index carbohydrates in the abovementioned study of teenage boys is in fact due to additional calorie intake. Thus I suggest eating high-fiber carbohydrates for their nutritional value and low calorie density, if there is credence to the theory that they help prevent excess calorie intake because of their lower glycemic index then all the better. This is just another reason to avoid processed carbohydrates.

Most people with insulin resistance don't go on to develop type 2 diabetes. Type 2 diabetes occurs only when insulin resistance results in a high blood sugar. What is critical for type 2 diabetics to understand is that by the time diabetes is diagnosed, the cells that normally secrete insulin in the pancreas (beta cells) have already started to fail. That is, as a result of the body's increasing insulin resistance, the beta cells can't produce enough insulin to keep the blood sugar normal. Therefore the usual course of type 2 diabetes is one of progressive beta cell failure and the eventual need for insulin administration to keep blood sugar in the normal range. With this in mind, let's discuss why *moderate* carbohydrate restriction in type 2 diabetes is appropriate. We will return to insulin resistance and its place as a target for treatment in type 2 diabetes later.

There are two different times metabolically during the day when a type 2 diabetic's blood sugar will be elevated. One is on awakening, before any food is eaten (doctors call this the fasting blood sugar), and before the other meals of the day. The second time is after eating a meal or snack (doctors call this the postprandial blood sugar). These blood sugars are high for two very different reasons. Fasting sugars are high primarily due to the inability of the pancreas to secrete enough insulin overnight to overcome insulin resistance at the liver. A normal liver is very sensitive to insulin overnight and shuts off sugar production and release so that the blood sugar is normal when we wake up. In diabetes the liver is resistant to insulin and continues to make and release sugar overnight, leading to a high blood sugar on awakening. This explains the perplexing phenomenon of going to sleep with a good blood sugar (for instance, after taking insulin before supper) and waking up the next morning with a high blood sugar.

On the other hand, postprandial blood sugar is high primarily because the pancreas is unable to produce enough insulin to keep the carbohydrates eaten during a meal from remaining in the bloodstream as sugar instead of passing into the body's cells. Although carbohydrate intake doesn't usually have much of a direct effect on the fasting blood sugar, it does have a direct effect on the postprandial blood sugar. This is why it is important for diabetics to restrict not just sugar intake but also carbohydrates. Carbohydrates are the primary cause of elevation in blood sugar after meals. Diabetics who restrict carbohydrates (for example, to 45 grams per meal) will be able to reduce their postprandial blood sugar. In my experience, moderate carbohydrate restriction (potentially a large change in a diet already rich in carbohydrates) may delay a patient's need to add additional diabetes drugs to keep blood sugar normal or delay the addition of insulin to oral drugs. Carbohydrate restriction will also help reduce calories and help with weight loss, which will indirectly improve blood sugar control by reducing insulin resistance. For diabetics, too, carbohydrates high in fiber are also preferable to refined carbohydrates.

There is no question that insulin shots cause weight gain through several different mechanisms. Insulin (and for that matter oral medication) improves blood sugar control, reducing the amount of sugar (and hence calories) lost in the urine. Patients also find themselves eating extra calories to prevent low blood sugar, with resultant weight gain. I see diabetic patients every day who have continued trouble with high blood sugar and therefore need to have their insulin doses increased. The result is more weight gain and further insulin resistance, resulting in a vicious cycle of more high blood sugars, further increases in insulin dosing, and therefore more weight gain. The way to break this cycle is to significantly reduce carbohydrate intake. Blood sugar after meals will inevitably come down, and the insulin dose can then be reduced. With reduction in insulin dose, a patient will have a much easier time losing the unwanted pounds. I must emphasize that this type of carbohydrate restriction should never be done without the direct supervision of a physician so that the insulin dose can be safely reduced. Coming off insulin completely once it has been started is the exception, as diabetics' pancreatic dysfunction is not reversible, but there are exceptions to the rule, such as recently diagnosed diabetics who are on small doses of insulin and/or lose a large amount of weight. Blood sugar control is critical, however, and the more common scenario is to wait too long to begin insulin therapy and not to be aggressive enough with insulin dosing once it has been instituted.

One more point regarding diabetes treatment: up until the mid-1990s in the United States, the only drugs that were available to treat diabetes were of the type that cause increased insulin secretion (glyburide, glipizide, etc.). With the introduction of metformin to the U.S. market, a drug that reduced insulin resistance became available. In the late 1990s a group of diabetes medications known as the thiazolidinediones or TZDs (now marketed as Actos and Avandia) became available. Unlike metformin, which is primarily an insulin sensitizer at the liver (with some fat and muscle insulin sensitization), TZDs reduce insulin resistance primarily at fat tissue and muscle. These two different classes of drugs address the insulin resistance syndrome in different ways.

Metformin as an initial therapy in obese diabetic patients in a large diabetes study in the United Kingdom reduced heart disease risk. This was independent of blood sugar control and was likely due to improving insulin resistance and its resultant effect on various heart disease risk factors.[6] Additionally, metformin does not cause weight gain. Actos and Avandia likely have the same type of heart disease risk reduction through different mechanisms, but long-term studies are still pending. Although the TZDs can cause weight gain, the fat gained is subcutaneous (under the skin), not in the abdominal area, and therefore does not worsen insulin resistance; in fact, as mentioned these drugs reduce insulin resistance. Not all patients will gain weight on TZDs. I've seen patients lose weight on these drugs with carbohydrate restriction. Given the improvement in insulin resistance afforded by these drugs and their probable heart disease benefit independent of blood sugar control, I believe that all type 2 diabetics should be on metformin or a TZD unless there is a contraindication. It is important to also note that these drugs have no risk of low blood sugar reactions if used alone. Therefore (with some exceptions, as will always be the case in medicine), I suggest *there should be no such thing as "diet-controlled" diabetes*. Even if blood sugar levels are almost normal, these drugs reduce insulin resistance, which is the core problem. In fact, future studies will likely show reduction in heart disease in patients with insulin resistance on these drugs even before they develop diabetes. And perhaps there will soon be newer drugs as well that will target insulin resistance without causing weight gain.

In summary, it is weight gain that causes elevated insulin levels, not the reverse. Moderate carbohydrate restriction in type 2 diabetics is important for its help with weight loss and to help prevent high blood sugar after meals. Carbohydrate restriction can also help diabetics on insulin reduce the amount of insulin they take and thereby help prevent or reverse the weight gain that occurs with high insulin dosing. Otherwise, although dramatic carbohydrate restriction or elimination causes weight loss through the resultant calorie restriction, it is not a maintainable option for weight loss. Weight regain will occur after the inevitable reintroduction of carbohydrates to the diet. Pancreatic insulin release in response to the ingestion of carbohydrates with a high glycemic index *may* have an indirect effect on weight gain by causing drops in blood sugar levels that result in hunger and spur overeating. This however remains an unproven hypothesis. We recommend high-fiber carbohydrates to avoid this potential obstacle specifically and for their nutritional benefit in general. High-fiber carbohydrates such as fruits and vegetables also tend to fill us up after fewer calories and help reduce total calorie intake. Otherwise, in my opinion, the glycemic index in and of itself is a complex and impractical tool for maintainable weight right now.

Chapter 5

THE BEHAVIORAL ASPECTS OF
WEIGHT LOSS AND GENERAL PREMISES
OF THE NANTUCKET DIET

*T*he Nantucket Diet presents a formula that sets dieters up for long-term success. The specifics of this formula and its implementation are reviewed in Chapters 6 and 7. Before you proceed, I want to review some guiding principles that will help with your transition to a healthier lifestyle. Some of the currently accepted behavioral modification techniques for weight loss fit nicely with our diet scheme and are discussed in this chapter.

There is no argument that Americans overeat. I propose that the solution to weight gain is addressing this habit of overeating and not promoting dramatic and unsustainable restriction of food intake. My clinical experience is that the patients who successfully lose and maintain their weight are those who make small but consistent changes in their *overeating habits,* not their eating habits. They achieve weight loss without hunger and do not see their changes as burdensome or obsessive.

It is this change in overeating habits and not in eating habits that I encourage. While this distinction may sound trivial, in fact very small changes in calorie intake result in significant weight gain or loss when dealing with the finely tuned metabolism of the human body. Small numbers of unnecessary calories at each meal add up over time to a large cumulative weight gain. By consciously avoiding these unnecessary extra calories you will reduce your daily calorie intake in a relatively painless manner. These unnecessary calories are those that come from large portions, from second and third helpings, and from eating so quickly that the body's signal of satiety (feeling full) is missed or ignored. Importantly, these are also the calories that come from eating calorie-dense foods—items that deliver many more calories for the same volume of food. You therefore want to pick foods that are less calorie-dense. Eating foods that are low in calorie density allows you to eat more food and to feel full after fewer calories.

Satiety or feeling full is your body's intrinsic overeating alarm. Learning to stop eating when full appears to be a very important skill for weight loss success. A recent study of premenopausal women looked at eating behaviors such as eating at bedtime, eating between meals, and eating beyond the point of feeling full, to see which of these is a risk factor for weight gain. In this study the only behavior that was correlated with an increase in weight was eating beyond feeling full.[1] Thus the extra calories eaten after our body tells us to stop seem to be a critical contributor to overeating and weight gain. If you are full . . . stop eating!

I deliberately used the term *skill* when referring to the ability to recognize when you are full and should stop eating. The experts teach us that behavioral approaches to weight loss should be process-oriented. This means learning the how-to of weight loss and not just choosing an end goal. Therefore it has been suggested that *the weight loss process should be viewed as a set of skills that need to be mastered, rather than the presence or absence of willpower.*[2] One such skill is listening to your body's signal to stop eating. With this in mind, let's discuss some of the key behavioral techniques or skills used in successful weight loss programs.

1. *Self-monitoring.* This is the cornerstone of dietary behavioral modification. Self-monitoring instruments such as diet logbooks help you uncover eating patterns that you were previously unaware of, and also reveal the tendency to underestimate calorie intake.[3] Obviously you need to be able to look back at your records and learn from your mistakes so that they are not repeated, so the records are useless unless you review them.

2. *Stimulus control.* This helps you avoid exposure to situations that lead to poor food choices. One example that has been given is avoiding high-risk venues such as fast-food restaurants.[4]

3. *Cognitive restructuring.* This is the process of eliminating self-destructive thoughts that result in behaviors that sabotage weight loss efforts. An example would be avoiding self-criticism after overeating. Such self-criticism leads to despair and hopelessness, which then result in further binge eating.[5] Obviously this reaction makes the problem worse. You should have a mechanism in place to deal emotionally with the occasional inevitable backslide.[6] You want a plan that prevents a minor indiscretion from turning into a major transgression. For instance, after overeating, learn to encourage yourself to get back on track at the next meal rather than giving up.

4. *Modification of your home environment.* Eliminate cues for overeating; suggestions have included exchanging the cookie jar for a fruit bowl.[7]

5. *Dealing with stress eating or comfort eating.* If you find yourself eating extra calories to deal subconsciously with stress, you will hinder any attempts at weight loss. This is a very common and difficult problem. To begin the process of solving this problem, you must first recognize that you are stress eating. Stop and ask yourself, Do I need to exercise restraint? Am I comfort eating? If the answer is yes, walk away from the food. You then need to identify the underlying stressor and address it either alone or with help. Ultimately the stressor must be dealt with directly to eliminate the symptom of stress eating.

In the meantime, you want to establish a readily accessible *personal behavioral dominion*—a territory in which you exercise complete behavioral control—to which you can escape to remove yourself from food and stress. This is a behavioral technique that requires a conscious effort and an understanding that it won't be easy. You want to engage in activities within this personal dominion that are incompatible with eating. For instance, don't read the paper at the breakfast room table. The following recommendations are just examples to help you establish a personal behavioral dominion that works for you. The key is that you consciously decide to remove yourself from the comfort food.

- Distance yourself from food; let sugarless gum keep your mouth busy.
- Maintain an ongoing project that you can return to on a routine basis and keeps your interest. This could be any home improvement project, yard work, learning a musical instrument, writing, or reading a novel.
- Listen to music no matter what your activity. There is no greater mood stabilizer in my opinion.
- Invest one-on-one time with your children; get down on the floor and give them your undivided attention.
- Return to nature. Walk the dog or exercise outdoors.
- Reestablish intimacy with your spouse or significant other. Talk or reinfuse some romance into your relationship. Replace comfort food with comfort romance!
- Get involved in a community organization. Keep an interest in life outside your home and let others benefit from your behavioral modification.
- Look into the local nightlife, go out and explore museums, etc.

All of the above activities require effort, as do all worthwhile endeavors. All are rewarding and achieve comfort-food avoidance. You know yourself best; pick an activity that you know will be distracting and promise yourself you'll make the effort to stick with it.

In addition to the above skills, I recommend that you begin the practice of separating your meals into courses. In other words, don't put out all the food at once. Put out one dish, eat, clear the table, and then bring out the next dish. This will slow down your eating and allow for your satiety signal to be appreciated, resulting in a lower calorie intake. It allows you to start meals with healthy foods such as salads and vegetables that should reduce the total number of calories per meal. It will also provide more time for your family to talk and for you to catch up and connect with your children. In fact, eating dinner as a family has in and of itself been associated with healthier food choices.[8] What is the downside to eating in courses? There will be more dishes to clean, and more time taken to eat in a busy world. If this is not realistic for all of your meals, then start doing it with three or four meals per week.

Even with the best behavioral techniques, you need to make wise food choices. For practical purposes, this means eating foods with less fat (fat has the highest calorie count per gram) and fewer processed carbohydrates (which are low in fiber and high in calorie density). It's nice to know that fat-restricted diets can cause a sensation of satiety, which will help you avoid the hunger pangs people fear. And if you think you are a fat addict, good news—it has been noted that people on diets high in fiber can eventually lose their attraction to high-fat foods.[9] I propose eating more bulky foods, such as fruits and vegetables, that are high in fiber. These are not calorie-dense and therefore will lead to a sensation of being full with less calorie consumption. In this way you can cut calories but continue to eat a reasonable volume of food, thereby avoiding the feeling of starvation and the obsession with food that many diets create. The dramatic changes in food intake fad diets propose can lead to constant hunger—you're always thinking about the next meal. Unlike other diets, the Nantucket Diet allows you to think of your daily routine between meals and not food. In fact, I recommend snacking. Snacking patterns are lifelong learned behaviors and extremely difficult to change. Snacking should be continued, but the types of snack food should be changed. Eating the same number of snacks but improving their quality will further reduce total daily calorie intake. I implore you to have one midmorning and one midafternoon snack to prevent hunger and the resultant desire to overeat at the next meal.

Therefore generally, I propose modest calorie reduction through avoidance of calorie-dense foods and through portion control. I recommend snacks, but with a change in the quality of your snacks so that premeal hunger is avoided. Specifically (don't worry, all the details of how to start and maintain your diet plan are coming up in the next chapter), I recommend reducing cumulative daily calories (total number of calories added together from all three meals and snacks) by 500 to 1,000 per day, depending on your starting weight. To put this into perspective, for some of you this will mean not much more than eliminating that large glass of OJ for breakfast (200 calories) and that nondiet 20-ounce soda at lunch (250 calories). By following these recommendations you can expect to lose one half to one pound per week.[10] There will be no initial dramatic weight loss. This rate of weight loss may seem slow at first glance but adds up to 25 to 50 pounds per year. The key here is that these lost pounds will be easier to keep off because the changes in diet are modest and sustainable. Understand that the pounds we gain are put on slowly, so we need to give a legitimate alteration in eating habits time to get these same pounds off. And unlike fad diets, these changes in diet are maintainable, so the pounds will stay off permanently.

The Nantucket Diet also *requires* one meal per week that will not be constrained by the diet's guidelines. People following fad diets have a lot of stored-up calorie desires that are released when the rigorous part of the diet is completed and a return to a more normal diet is attempted. This inevitably results in overindulgence in high-calorie foods. If a dieter knows it's OK to stray from the diet at the end of each week, this "cheating" energy is released a little at a time, so there is no dramatic buildup resulting in binge eating behavior. Life is short, and I understand that dieters want to enjoy some culinary pleasures. I call this designated unrestricted meal each week the Make Love to Life meal. This meal has no specific limitations and may include anything you desire, such as a decadent dessert.

Remember that although it is quantity of food that determines weight loss, the quality of food is important for overall health. I recognize that certain types of carbohydrates and fats, in addition to high calorie density, have independent detrimental health effects—for instance, on cholesterol levels—and I have made specific recommendations in this regard in Chapter 3. These recommendations fit nicely into the type of diet plan already discussed because foods low in fat and high in fiber, such as fruits and vegetables, are not only heart-healthy but low in calorie density as well. Thus these foods have a double benefit. The type of food you choose in general—for example, a Mediterranean-style diet as discussed in Chapter 3—is your preference. I want you to eat foods you like.

The Nantucket Diet's recommendations are backed by the current scientific literature. Recently published data by the U.S. Department of Agriculture reveal that lifestyle modification results in sustained weight loss, whereas fad diets do not. In keeping with this philosophy, NIH weight loss guidelines recommend modest calorie restriction for slow and sustained weight loss. These guidelines are the ones we have chosen to promote to ensure the Nantucket Diet is a practical and effective path to permanent weight loss and total health.

As might be expected, diet is not the only tool for weight loss. Exercise is critical for weight loss and maintenance and is complementary to diet. Not only will exercise alone result in weight loss independent of diet, but diet combined with exercise results in more weight loss than either component alone.[11] Physical activity is also important during weight loss to help maintain lean body mass.[12] Surprisingly, even minimal activity such as fidgeting has been shown to contribute to weight loss.[13] In addition, exercise contributes to improved cardiac and pulmonary fitness independent of weight loss.[14] That is, exercise has a direct beneficial effect on the heart and lungs that is not related to weight loss alone. Exercise also improves insulin resistance both immediately and in the long term. There should also be no doubt that your general sense of well-being is improved with exercise and that there is a tremendous sense of accomplishment as the body's strength and endurance improve with a regular exercise regimen.

You should view your exercise as you do your checkbook. Exercise will tip your daily net calorie balance to weight loss. Calories burned will contribute to weight loss or will allow you to eat more daily calories if you are in a weight maintenance phase. The formula provided to you for your daily calorie needs therefore will take exercise into account. So not only does exercise benefit your heart, it allows you to be a little more liberal with your calories.

Please know I am not trying to pull the wool over your eyes. Weight loss is not always easy. To suggest anything else would be dishonest. The guidelines set forth in this book are only tools and need to be implemented consistently to work. If you are like many of our readers, you have lost weight in the past but have been frustrated when the pounds were regained. Commitment to a long-term lifestyle modification will be needed to give you the best chance for weight loss and maintenance. Several motivating factors have been identified that contribute to the successful implementation of weight loss programs. Among these are a good understanding of obesity and its health risks, good social support from friends and family, and a good attitude toward physical activity and the willingness to take time to participate in it.[15] I strongly encourage you to get the above motivators in place before starting your lifestyle modification to give yourself the best chance for success. Reinforcement of these motivators as you lose weight is a sound policy. Going into this program with a partner, although not necessary, is strongly recommended to help maintain good motivation. Once the pounds start to come off, you'll establish some weight loss momentum, and this in itself will be motivation for further weight loss. Contrary to what you might think, weighing yourself frequently has been shown to be associated with successful weight loss, probably due to this type of motivation.

It is also worth pointing out that even the most motivated individual is subject to temptation. It is critical that you adjust your shopping habits. Make a shopping list and stick to it. Don't browse down the high-calorie aisles. All calorie-dense food should be removed from the home at the start of the Nantucket Diet. This includes sweets, processed and packaged foods high in calories and saturated or trans fats, and anything that would come under the heading of junk food. Get rid of all the nondiet sodas, ice cream, and high-calorie juices. Get rid of the desserts. If they are not in the house, you won't be tempted to pull them out of the pantry at 10 p.m. Family members should respect your need to avoid these items. If they must have them in the house, ask that they shop for them themselves (that should put that issue to rest) and keep them in a separate place away from your food.

The many easy-to-prepare, healthy, and delicious recipes included in this book will certainly help smooth the transition to a healthy diet. These recipes, as the title of our book suggests, are steeped in Nantucket and New England culinary culture and include a large number of contributions from some of the finest restaurants on Nantucket. Eating healthy food doesn't mean eating food that doesn't taste good. We understand that people want to eat food they enjoy, and this is the driving force of *The Nantucket Diet*'s extensive recipe section.

Chapter 6

GETTING STARTED: THE FORMULA

*T*he following pages introduce you to the formula that is the foundation of the Nantucket Diet. I will help you use this formula to calculate your daily calorie needs at the end of this chapter. Once done, you can proceed to Chapter 7, which lays out the three phases of our diet plan.

Changing dietary habits should be likened to studying. The hardest part is just getting started. Once you have begun the process, things will fall into place. Set a start date and be sure to keep it. Get your environment in order. There is no need to surround yourself with unnecessary temptation. You wouldn't expect someone with a history of alcoholism to have much success avoiding alcohol in a bar. Likewise, a kitchen full of junk food makes it next to impossible to resist eating calorie-dense foods, whether for dessert or at midnight. I therefore would like to reemphasize that your shopping habits must change. Shopping at the supermarket must be deliberate and organized. If you don't buy junk food, you won't eat it. If you have any junk food left in your home, get rid of it. Let the people you work with know that you are trying to avoid junk food, so they won't offer it to you. Don't be self-conscious. Your coworkers are likely to show an interest in your diet plan and join you. The more support you have at home and at work, the easier your lifestyle changes will be.

As you read the specifics of the Nantucket Diet and begin its implementation, keep the following tips in mind:

WEIGHT LOSS TIPS, A TO Z

A. Shop wisely. If you don't buy it, you won't try it!

B. Although weight loss occurs through calorie reduction and exercise, don't forget the principles discussed in Chapter 3 regarding the types and quality of the food you eat. Eat foods low in calorie density so that you will get more food volume for the same number of calories and feel full when done with a meal. Eat foods high in fiber and low in trans and saturated fats to derive the health benefits these foods offer.

C. Purchase low-calorie versions of your favorite foods, such as low-fat cheese or skim milk. As an example, a cup of whole milk is 150 calories, but a cup of skim milk is only 90 calories.

D. Stay within your daily calorie goal. The calories can be divided into meals and snacks in any way you wish.

E. Plan your meals when possible, the most important likely being lunch at work. You don't want to put yourself in the position of having to eat pepperoni pizza at the office because you didn't prepare an alternative meal. I know it's easier not to think about what you eat, but those days unfortunately are over or you wouldn't be reading this book.

F. Never skip a meal. If you skip meals, you will inevitably overeat at subsequent meals.

G. Eat slowly so you can exploit your body's built-in satiety mechanism (the signal that tells you when you are full).

H. Eat a healthy, low-calorie snack such as fruit, vegetables, or nuts midmorning and midafternoon every day to avoid unnecessary hunger. This allows you to concentrate on your life and not obsess about food.

I. It has been shown that a healthy salad at the beginning of a meal reduces total calorie intake.[1] I recommend trying to eat one or two salads per day for this reason as well as for the healthy fiber and other nutrients salads provide. Add dressings that are low-calorie. Don't weigh the salad down with a high-calorie, high-fat dressing.

J. Remember that you are *required* to eat one meal per week that is without dietary constraint. I call this the Make Love to Life meal. It's unrealistic to expect complete elimination of any specific foods, and it's nice to know you can "cheat" once per week. Life is too short to deprive yourself of culinary pleasures.

K. Avoid wasting calories on beverages. Drink water, flavored sparkling water, or diet beverages. Add a slice of lemon or lime to your water. Drink at least three to four glasses of water or other noncaloric beverage per day.

L. If you are raiding the fridge for something cold like ice cream, popsicles, or fruit, you may be mistaking thirst for hunger. The tip-off here is the drive to ingest something *cold*. Consider this possibility and have a cold calorie free beverage. You may surprise yourself.

M. Don't waste calories on cream and sugar in your coffee. Use skim milk and artificial sweetener. Recent data reveals a reduced risk of diabetes as a fringe benefit of coffee drinking.[2] Don't overdo it, however, as too much coffee can worsen high blood pressure and cause heart symptoms such as palpitations.

N. Don't make fast food a habit. Fast food is a prime example of calorie-dense food, discussed in Chapter 5. A little fast food delivers a tremendous number of calories—exactly what I am suggesting you try to avoid. A fast-food meal provides over twice the calories needed for a healthy diet. When eating fast food, we inadvertently engage in what has been labeled "passive overconsumption."[3] This is a wonderfully descriptive term. We can pack away a tremendous number of calories with fast food, we don't have to work to do it, and because of the calorie density of fast food our bodies don't realize we've overeaten. Fast food can also contain high-risk fats contributing to heart disease and may have few redeeming nutrients.

O. Don't eat snacks or meals in front of the TV. This leads to grazing and hundreds of unnecessary calories.

P. Don't eat the leftovers on your kid's plate at the end of a meal.

Q. Try olive or canola oil sprays for your cooking. These sprays are quite tasty and have only a few calories. Although their labels will say zero calories, check out the serving size (listed as duration of spray)—the spray I have labels a serving size as one-third of a second, which seems a little silly. The amount you will more typically use probably has a few calories, but it is certainly going to be far fewer than butter or margarine. If you must use butter, select the lite/whipped variety, which has about two-thirds fewer calories.

R. Try a plant stanol margarine such as Benecol® or Take Control® in place of butter if you have high cholesterol. Stanol margarine has just over half the calories of butter and has been shown to reduce LDL (bad) cholesterol by 10 to 20 percent.[4]

S. Use fat-free chicken or vegetable broth in place of oils in gravy and sauces to get more flavor for fewer calories.

T. If you are a diabetic and find yourself frequently eating snacks to treat or prevent low blood sugar, consult your physician. These extra calories make weight loss more difficult. With the newer diabetes drugs and insulins now available, your diabetic regimen should be tailored to your lifestyle, not the reverse.

U. If you are a diabetic on insulin and not restricting your carbohydrate intake, talk to your physician. Reducing your carbohydrate intake will lower your postprandial blood sugar and enable your physician to decrease your insulin dose. In addition to taking in fewer calories in the form of carbohydrates, you will have an easier time losing weight on less insulin. Do this only under direct physician supervision to avoid low blood sugar reactions.

V. Grill, don't fry. Remember not to eat any charred areas to avoid potential carcinogens.

W. Eat lean meats, fish, and poultry.

X. Assuming you have no personal history of alcoholism and are a current drinker, I recommend one glass of wine several times per week at your evening meal. We provide wine recommendations with many of our dinner recipes. The potential health benefits of moderate alcohol consumption have already been reviewed in Chapter 3.

Y. Buy a pedometer and use it to measure the number of miles you walk per day. Your pedometer will give you an idea of how you are progressing with your exercise program. There is actually data suggesting that using a pedometer leads to increased exercise, probably because it serves as a motivator.[5]

Z. Burn extra calories through exercise on the day you eat your Make Love to Life meal.

YOUR TOTAL ENERGY EXPENDITURE (TEE)

Let's now proceed to your weight loss formula. The first component of the Nantucket Diet is an equation that serves as the foundation for your calorie manipulation and gives you the ability to regain control of your energy balance. This equation determines your Total Energy Expenditure, or TEE. Your TEE represents the calories needed to maintain your current weight at your current activity level. Although you obviously don't want to maintain your current weight, your TEE will be used as a dynamic individualized starting point from which you will achieve consistent weight loss. The TEE is a combination of two formulas that were derived by scientists over the last century. When applied in creative ways to each of the Nantucket Diet's three phases of weight control, the TEE becomes a powerful (as well as fun, believe it or not) tool for weight loss success. As you will see, the TEE allows for a weight loss program tailored to your individual calorie needs. You don't need to worry about complicated math. All formulas are provided in straightforward and simple terms. If you choose (as we suggest), you can use the calculators found on our Web site, www.nantucketdiet.com, for instantaneous results.

The first half of your TEE is your Basal Energy Expenditure, also called basal metabolic rate. The Basal Energy Expenditure formula was derived in the early twentieth century by two scientists named J. Arthur Harris and Francis G. Benedict.[6] The formula is therefore often referred to as the Harris-Benedict equation. Your Basal Energy Expenditure is a determination of the energy you expend, measured in calories, to maintain all of your body's functions while at rest. It takes into account your weight, height, age, and gender to determine the number of calories needed to maintain your current weight. This formula is well known in the nutrition community and is used by nutritionists in hospitals to determine sick patients' calorie needs so that lean body mass is not lost and patients have adequate nutrition to fight off illness. As it turns out, the formula is quite handy outside the hospital to determine calories needed to lose weight. The Basal Energy Expenditure will allow you to manipulate your calorie intake to achieve weight loss as you proceed with the Nantucket Diet. Although it is clearly an estimate, a recent review of Harris and Benedict's formula suggests that it is valid and widely applicable.[7] I am not suggesting that the Basal Energy Expenditure can be used to dial calories up or down to the exact pound, but your Basal Energy Expenditure, when used as a part of your TEE, will provide you with the tool you need to regain control of your body's weight changes. I provide the Basal Energy Expenditure formula here in the book, or you can simply go to our Web site and plug your weight, height, gender, and age into the calculator and see your Basal Energy Expenditure result instantaneously. As you lose weight your Basal Energy Expenditure will change and you will be able to quickly recalculate it to help adjust calorie intake as you proceed. For simplicity's sake, I am going to call the Basal Energy Expenditure your Resting Metabolism.

Note that the calorie requirements estimated using the formula for Resting Metabolism will be significantly higher for men than women because men have more lean body mass. Therefore men will likely have an easier time than women losing weight because of their generally higher percentage of lean body mass. Let's take the example of two thirty-nine-year-old people, each weighing 170 pounds at 5 feet 8 inches. One is a man and one a woman. When their numbers are plugged into the Resting Metabolism equation, the man can eat 1,728 calories and maintain his weight, whereas the woman can eat only 1,531 calories if she wishes to maintain her weight (not taking any activity into account). Looked at another way, if the man ate 1,531 calories, he'd lose weight, whereas the woman would theoretically not lose a pound. Not fair. This is why exercise can be a wonderful ally for women. If the same woman burns 200 calories per day with exercise, she will level the playing field.

As you might expect, your total daily calorie requirements depend not just on your Resting Metabolism but on how active you are and therefore how many additional calories are burned as a result of this activity. The second part of your Total Energy Expenditure is an adjustment factor related to your level of physical activity. This adjustment factor, called your Physical Activity Level (PAL), is then multiplied by your Resting Metabolism. Your PAL is determined using a simple chart we provide. This PAL chart is based on researchers' estimates of physical activity measured in calories. Thus by multiplying your Resting Metabolism by your Physical Activity Level, your final Total Energy Expenditure result is obtained.[8] Remember, the TEE is the number of calories, at your current weight and activity level, that you can eat to maintain your current weight. The TEE will be applied to each phase of the Nantucket Diet, as you will soon see.

Let's go ahead and calculate your TEE. As you know, your TEE is calculated by multiplying your Resting Metabolism by your PAL. There are four simple steps that we will guide you through below (you should pull out your calculator for these calculations), or you can use the TEE calculator on our Web site. We provide an example on the next page to help make things easier.

STEP 1 FOR MEN:
Estimated Resting Metabolism is calculated as follows:
> **66.5 + (6.25 × weight in pounds) + (12.7 × height in inches) − (6.755 × age in years)**

STEP 1 FOR WOMEN:
Estimated Resting Metabolism is calculated as follows:
> **655 + (4.35 × weight in pounds) + (4.69 × height in inches) − (4.67 × age in years)**

STEP 2:
Next multiply the Resting Metabolism result just calculated by .95. (The Harris-Benedict equation may overestimate Resting Metabolism by 5 percent or more. We therefore ask that you subtract 5 percent from your Resting Metabolism—hence multiplying by .95—so that you favor weight loss if there is an overestimation.)[9] Write this number down.

Here's an example.

A thirty-nine-year-old woman is 5 feet 8 inches tall and weighs 175 pounds.

655 + (4.35 × 175 pounds) + (4.69 × 68 inches) − (4.67 × 39 years)

655 + 761.25 + 319 − 182 = 1,553

1553 × .95 = 1475

Thus 1,475 is the estimated Resting Metabolism for this woman.

STEP 3: SELECT YOUR PAL

Because the PAL is only an estimate and because of significant variation in published PAL ranges,[10, 11, 12] I have listed a Nantucket Diet PAL chart that represents what I believe to be a conservative approach to PAL determination. The PAL catagories below will hedge your bet to favor weight loss rather than risking an overestimation of your PAL.

PHYSICAL ACTIVITY LEVEL (PAL) ESTIMATES	
1.1	sedentary or immobilized
1.40	minimal activity*
1.55	moderate activity (exercise, walking, etc., an average of 30 minutes most days)†
1.75	very active (running 30 plus minutes three or more times per week)‡

*above activity is in addition to your normal activities of daily living
†if activity falls between two levels you can split the difference, e.g., PAL of 1.65
‡If you can't decide between two categories, choose the lower of the two e.g. 1.55 vs. 1.75; choose 1.55.

RESTING METABOLISM × PAL = YOUR TEE

STEP 4:

Multiply Resting Metabolism result from Step 2 by selected PAL.

Congratulations! You have just calculated your current Total Energy Expenditure. As you will see in the next chapter, this one number will be the basis for your successful navigation through the three phases of the Nantucket Diet.

Chapter 7

THE NANTUCKET DIET'S
THREE PHASES

*T*he Nantucket Diet consists of three phases. As you proceed through each phase, you will use your newly calculated TEE as a powerful weight loss tool. In Phase 1 you will terminate weight gain. In Phase 2 you will lose weight at a healthy, consistent pace. When you have reached your goal weight, you will enter Phase 3 to maintain your newly achieved weight loss. As you will see, all three phases provide flexibility and can be customized to your specific needs.

Phase 1
TERMINATION OF WEIGHT GAIN

If you are like most Americans, you are not just overweight but progressively gaining weight as the years go by. Therefore, your first goal is to terminate this weight gain and establish your current weight as your *launch weight*. Your launch weight is your Nantucket Diet starting weight. We therefore call the TEE you just calculated in Chapter 6 your *launch weight TEE*—these are

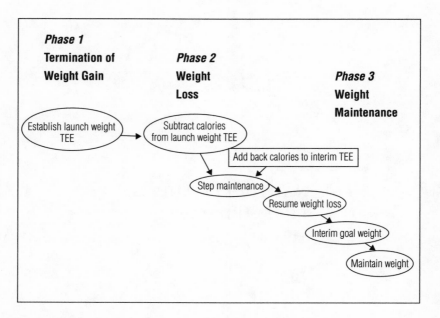

the calories needed just to maintain your launch weight and not continue to gain. You will now log your current daily calorie intake and compare this to your launch weight TEE.

I believe it is helpful to add up the calories per day you are currently eating for two reasons. (1) It is important to appreciate the difference between your current calorie intake and your launch weight TEE calories. This difference represents the calories beyond those your body needs to maintain its current weight, and these extra calories result in weight gain. Calculating the difference between your current calorie intake and your launch weight TEE should give you an appreciation of just how much you are overeating. (2) This is also an opportunity to learn tricks for easy calorie counting (discussed later in more detail). You can use package labels, or search the USDA Nutrient Database (go to www.nal.usda.gov/fnic/foodcomp/index.html and click on Download Software) that is downloadable from the Internet to your computer or PDA (calories are listed as "energy-Kcal"). As a result of food labeling requirements and technology such as the ability to search the USDA's database of 6,800 different food items, there has never been an easier time to count calories. Take advantage of your PDA and computer. It's the sedentary lifestyle we've developed as a result of technology that's gotten us into this weight gain dilemma, so it's nice to be able to exploit technology to help make losing the weight a little easier.

STEP **1** *How Many Calories Are You Currently Eating?* Carefully add up the total daily calories for all of your meals and snacks for each of four consecutive days. Be sure to include two weekend days. Once done, add all four days' calories together and divide by four. This will give you your current daily calorie intake. You can plug your calories into our Web site calculator at www.nantucketdiet.com, and get your current daily calorie intake instantaneously if you wish. This calorie average is what has been responsible for your weight gain. And it is this weight gain that you will terminate. *Please do not change your diet during these four days, and include all calories to assure a fair caloric estimation.*

STEP **2** *How Many Calories Are You Overeating Each Day?* Subtract your launch weight TEE from your current daily calorie intake just calculated in step 1. As an example, if your current average is 2,500 calories per day and your launch weight TEE is 2,000 calories per day, then you subtract 2,000 from 2,500. The resulting 500 calories in this example are the calories you are eating beyond your launch weight TEE. These are the calories that will need to be eliminated to terminate your weight gain and maintain your launch weight.

STEP **3** *Terminate Weight Gain.* Eat the calories that add up to your launch weight TEE for one to two weeks. This will maintain your launch weight during that time. This period will help you slowly adjust to your new lifestyle changes and get you through Phase 1 with relative ease. This is your first step in regaining control of your weight. If after checking with your doctor you slowly begin an exercise program during Phase 1, you may in fact lose weight. The calories burned through exercise will bring your net daily calorie count below your launch weight TEE and therefore contribute to weight loss.

You can distribute your total daily calories across your meals and snacks in any way you wish. It's critical only that you have three meals and two snacks, as discussed previously. If you are eager to get on with weight loss, you may wish to limit Phase 1 to one week. This is not unreasonable, but I do advise the full two weeks for Phase 1 if your launch weight TEE is more than 500 calories less than your current daily calorie intake. You want to undergo a gradual reduction in calories so your body has an easy transition into your new lifestyle.

Before I proceed to Phase 2, I'd like to give you a few tips on calorie counting. First and most important, there is no need to calculate to the exact calorie. Coming close should suffice. There are many ways to approach this. A visit with a nutritionist can help but is not necessary for our weight loss program. Calorie counts are present on prepackaged items at the supermarket and may be all you need to estimate your calorie intake. Remember not to be fooled by the serving size when recording your calories. The products you buy at the supermarket list calories per serving, not per package. Thus if there are three servings in a package, you will eat three times the calories listed if you eat the entire package of food. Oftentimes the manufacturer will consider a serving to be a good deal smaller than you would, and they are able to make their product look healthier by doing this. Additionally, don't be fooled by labels claiming a product is "low-fat." You may in fact consume a higher number of calories from the carbohydrates and sugar that are substituted for the fat in these products.

Nutrition Facts

Serving Size: 1/3 DANISH-2 OZ (57 g)
Servings Per Container: 12

Amount Per Serving

Calories 230   Calories from Fat 110

The label above is an example of a confusing calorie count. It was taken off a package containing four danish.

The calories are listed in bold print as 230 (almost half of which are from fat). However, if you eat one danish, you have actually eaten 230 × 3 or 690 calories! If you look closely at the serving size, it is listed as one-third of a danish.

Nantucket Dieter, *beware!*

Let us help you. All of our recipes have their calories and nutrient content listed, so you can easily include these calories in your daily total. In addition, the Nantucket Diet Meal Planner provides you with a large variety of meals and permits spontaneity of food choice, something that is often lacking in diet plans. We have included a calorie counter for you in addition to the link to the USDA's full online calorie and nutrient counter. As mentioned previously, this is quite complete and helpful even for the more experienced cooks among our readers. The USDA calorie counter can be downloaded to your desktop for searches and can also be downloaded to your PDA for a mobile reference. We highly recommend this. Brand names are included in the USDA counter, and calorie counts can be looked up for many national restaurant chains on the Internet as well. Never has it been easier to bring food to the office and maintain your diet plan.

Phase 2
WEIGHT LOSS

You are now beginning Phase 2 of the Nantucket Diet. To this point you have maintained your launch weight for one to two weeks by reducing your calorie intake to your launch weight TEE. Now it's time to lose weight. As described in Chapter 1, current weight loss guidelines recommend achievable rates of weight loss that are least likely to set the dieter up for failure or weight regain. That is, the quicker weight is lost, the more likely it is the result of an unsustainable alteration in diet. Weight lost quickly is more likely to be regained when the dieter is ultimately unable to maintain these dramatic dietary changes. Given this, and given data that show medical benefit from as little as a 5 to 10 percent weight loss, the National Institutes of Health proposes one half to one pound per week as the goal rate of weight loss for an initial weight loss of 10 percent over six months.[1] I subscribe to this philosophy and encourage you to speak not in terms of an ultimate goal weight but in terms of interim goal weights, each interim goal weight being 10 percent less than the preceding weight. So your initial interim goal weight should be 10 percent less than your launch weight. After the initial 10 percent weight loss has been achieved, further weight loss (another 10 percent) can be pursued. To achieve a 10 percent weight loss in six months you will need to reduce calorie intake below your launch weight TEE by 500–1,000 calories per day—the exact amount depends on your starting body mass index (BMI). If you didn't calculate your BMI when reading Chapter 1, then now is the time (see the table on page 6). People with a higher BMI will need to reduce their intake by a greater number of calories because the absolute number of pounds that represents a 10 percent weight loss is higher. For example, 10 percent of 350 pounds is 10 pounds more than 10 percent of 250 pounds and thus requires more calorie reduction.

FOR A BMI UP TO 35: SUBTRACT 500 CALORIES PER DAY FROM YOUR LAUNCH WEIGHT TEE TO ACHIEVE ONE HALF TO ONE POUND WEIGHT LOSS PER WEEK.

FOR A BMI ABOVE 35: SUBTRACT 750–1,000 CALORIES PER DAY FROM YOUR LAUNCH WEIGHT TEE TO ACHIEVE ONE TO TWO POUNDS WEIGHT LOSS PER WEEK.

I don't advise cutting calories beyond this 500–1,000 per day because it will be difficult to maintain. Although weight loss will theoretically be faster by cutting calories beyond 1,000 per day, it will be more likely regained. It's also not healthy to cut calories too dramatically. Don't starve yourself. If your calories per day in Phase 2 fall under 1,100, recheck your math; if the figure is correct, consult your physician before proceeding.

Let's take the example of a fifty-five-year-old man who weighs 220 pounds and is 5 feet 6 inches tall. His BMI is 35.6. If he loses 10 percent of his body weight in six months, he now weighs 198 pounds. This is approximately one pound lost per week for a total of 22 pounds in 6 months. He has broken the 200-pound mark and has reduced his BMI to 32. He has met his initial interim weight loss goal. This is a respectable achievement, and he has obtained significant health benefits. The changes made were not extreme and are maintainable. If another 10 percent loss is desired, the current weight loss plan can be continued. In fact, he is on the way to getting his BMI under 30, which takes him out of the obesity category completely and puts him into the overweight category. This is in stark contrast to a scenario where he tries to quickly get to an unachievable weight, such as his high school graduation weight. Not only would he set himself up for failure, but even if he came close to this unrealistic goal the dietary changes needed would not be maintainable, and he would regain all the weight in six to twelve months.

Step Maintenance Thus to this point Phase 2 of the Nantucket Diet involves subtracting the necessary calories from your Launch Weight TEE to achieve a 10 percent weight loss in six-month intervals as you proceed through your interim goal weights. Although guidance from the Meal Planner and our recipes will make this a relatively easy and maintainable phase, I understand that weight loss is a long-term commitment and that our readers aren't machines. I know that the best weight loss intentions will often come up against obstacles, both expected and unexpected. We have all seen friends and patients who work hard to lose weight, only to go on a ten-day cruise and regain all their lost pounds.

By applying the TEE to a technique I call *step maintenance,* I provide an innovative solution to this unfortunate and frustrating phenomenon.

Through step maintenance, you will be able to give yourself a break from Phase 2 weight loss while involved in any of life's pleasures and not lose the ground you've worked so hard to gain. Step maintenance once again involves the use of the TEE to regain control of your energy balance. Let's continue with our example of a cruise vacation. The day before you fly to Florida you will calculate your new TEE (using the same TEE formula on page 55) for that precruise weight and activity level. This precruise TEE is the number of calories you can eat per day to *maintain* that precruise weight and avoid weight regain. You will then increase your daily calorie intake (from the calories calculated to provide phase 2 weight loss) to this precruise TEE to maintain the weight loss that you had recently achieved. In this way you remain in control of your weight. You have chosen to enjoy the food on the cruise and allow yourself additional calories, but you know how many additional calories you can afford without risking regaining the weight you've already lost. You can then go back to weight loss when you return home. You resume weight loss by again subtracting the requisite number of calories (as you did on page 61) from your TEE after your cruise. Step maintenance will come in handy for many of life's events for which we may want to allow ourselves a few extra calories, such as the winter holidays, school finals week, and various types of vacations.

As you continue to lose weight in Phase 2 you will want to recalculate your TEE for every 15 pounds lost. As you might expect, the original TEE calculation you made will not apply once significant weight is lost. You want to stay on top of your calorie requirements. You will see your calorie requirements change as you lose weight and (we hope) increase your exercise.

Note: Exercise beyond that used to calculate your TEE will burn additional calories. You should monitor your exercise time, and you can then add these calories burned through exercise back to your food intake to keep your net calorie reduction as desired in Phase 2 weight loss. We provide an extensive list of calories burned per hour for various exercises and activities on page 267. Other lists can be found on the Internet as well. As an example, if you want to reduce your daily calorie intake in Phase 2 by 500 calories and you are burning an additional 250 calories per day with a new walking program, you can subtract the 250 calories burned from the 500 and therefore only have to reduce your food calories by 250 per day. Alternatively, you can keep your caloric intake the same and let the additional calories burned contribute to faster weight loss. Again, this is not going to be dialable to the exact pound. Everyone's body is different, so you will need to see how your body responds initially.

Phase 3
WEIGHT MAINTENANCE

This is the last of the three phases. You will have the independence to choose when to stop Phase 2 and go on to Phase 3 based on your chosen interim goal weight. As the name suggests, you are now at a final or interim goal weight and want to maintain your weight loss. Data from the National Weight Control Registry suggests that the longer you keep the weight off, the easier weight maintenance becomes. To achieve Phase 3 maintenance you want to calculate your TEE (at the weight you will be maintaining) and eat this number of calories per day to maintain your goal weight at that current activity level. The eating and exercise habits you have developed in Phases 1 and 2 will serve you well for weight maintenance in Phase 3. I hope Phase 3 is seen as a lifestyle maintenance phase so that you can reap the benefits of your weight loss indefinitely. The role exercise plays in weight maintenance can't be emphasized enough. You must make a conscious effort to keep your exercise plan in full gear. The calories you burn with exercise will offset calories taken in and when exercise dwindles, weight will be regained. I'll mention again that exercise is also worthwhile for its benefits beyond weight loss and maintenance including reduced insulin resistance, improved heart health, and general sense of well-being.

Note: All three phases can be reentered as desired, depending on where you are in your weight loss progress. If you have been maintaining a specific weight in Phase 3, you can decide at any time to lose more weight. To do this, you simply calculate your new TEE and subtract the requisite number of calories (page 55) to lose another 10 percent of your weight in 6 months, thereby leaving Phase 3 and returning to Phase 2. If you regain some weight (we are only human, after all) at some point down the road, you should go back to Phase 1 to terminate weight gain and then proceed to Phase 2 two weeks thereafter. In this way the three phases of the Nantucket Diet can be called on at any time to control your body weight and not let it control you.

PLANNING MEALS

There are two general options for meal and snack planning on our program. Each has its advantages and will suit different people and different situations. Both can be used by the same person. In addition, the recipes on the following pages are designed to help you plan and prepare good healthy food, and fit into both meal planning options.

1. Plan your own meals and snacks. This is certainly a viable option for everyone and of course should be your ultimate goal. The USDA Nutrient Database and package labeling can be easily used to estimate calories per serving. This option obviously provides the most independence. Our Web site is set up to help you keep track of your daily calories.

2. We present the Nantucket Diet Meal Planner in Chapter 8. Our Meal Planner provides meal and snack templates with variation based on daily calorie count. Any recipe or food item of equal calorie count can be interchanged, providing hundreds of options.

TROUBLESHOOTING

Not losing weight? Look to see if any of the pitfalls below apply, and try my recommended correction.

- **Don't weigh yourself for the first two weeks of Phase 2.** At one half to one pound per week, weight loss over the first two to three weeks of the Nantucket Diet may be difficult to appreciate for several reasons, including inaccurate scales and normal daily weight fluctuations that include things such as water weight changes.

- **Scale accuracy?** Get an accurate scale and make sure your scale is set to read zero when you are not on it. Weigh yourself without clothes first thing in the morning.

- **Trouble with motivation.** Get a partner to go on your diet program with you, reassess motivators as described in Chapter 5, and make weight loss a priority. Avoid temptation; get rid of any junk food left in your home.

- **Calculating error when calculating TEE.** Recalculate your TEE. Are you overestimating your Physical Activity Level when using the equation?

- **Error estimating number of daily calories you are eating.** Remember to be sure you know serving size, and register calories per serving when reading labels. It has been shown that people trying to lose weight tend to underestimate their calorie intake.[2] These unaccounted-for calories will slow weight loss.

- **Eating beyond your calculated TEE.** Any calories beyond your launch weight TEE or calculated Phase 2 daily calorie intake will prevent weight loss. Try changing snack quality and quantity. Maybe you need to save more calories for a specific meal, such as supper. Some people simply need to eat more at supper because it's a social meal with the family and helps avoid late-night snacking. Remember to eat a salad at the start of meals to help reduce hunger and limit calories.

- **Check your Phase 2 daily calorie intake.** Your daily intake for weight loss during Phase 2 should be at least 500 calories less than the original daily calorie intake you calculated in step 1 of Phase 1 (termination of weight loss) at the beginning of this chapter.

- **No exercise.** Start an exercise program with your physician's permission.

- **Diabetes and insulin dose.** If you are on insulin, talk to your doctor about reducing your carbohydrate intake so that he or she can safely reduce your insulin to help you get the upper hand with weight loss.

- **Diabetes and snacks.** If you have diabetes and are eating excess calories in the form of snacks to keep your blood sugar up, consult your physician.

- **Have your doctor review your medications.** Many (some seizure medications, depression and other psychiatric medications, and steroids such as prednisone, among others) can make it harder to lose weight. *Never stop a medication without discussing it with your doctor first.*

- **Ask your doctor if there is a need to check for unusual causes of resistance to weight loss.** Hypothyroidism is not uncommon, but things such as Cushing's syndrome (overproduction of cortisol) are far less likely.

- **Fluid retention.** Make sure you are having no problems with fluid retention if you have heart disease and/or are on diuretics (water pills).

- **Resistant metabolism.** Subtract 10 percent from your current TEE and reenter Phase 2. If you need to do this one or two times to get jump-started, you certainly can. You can also consider using one of the prescription medications currently on the market for weight loss under your physician's guidance. Remember, specific criteria must be met to be a candidate for one of these medications, and these drugs do have potential side effects that need to be reviewed. You should be on a calorie-restricted diet in any event when you start one of these medications, as you'll have a better chance of losing weight on the drugs—they aren't magic and work best when combined with diet and exercise. Plus, if you don't lose weight on the drugs, your insurance plan won't pay for a refill. I have to say that although these drugs have been shown (through different mechanisms) to help with weight loss, my experience prescribing them to patients in obesity referral visits is that the drugs can have side effects that limit their use. In addition, they can be very difficult to get cleared by certain insurance plans, which is frustrating for patients and doctors. Finally, the people who lose weight on the drugs are the ones who make the appropriate dietary changes in any event and would probably lose weight even without the drug. There is also a significant risk of weight regain when the drugs are discontinued.

- **Stress eating.** If you are eating to help yourself deal with depression or anxiety, you need to address the underlying problem before you will be successful with weight loss (see page 43).

- **Boredom.** If you are eating because you are bored, you need to find something else to do with your time, such as exercise.

- **Calorie intake below 1,100.** As noted previously, if your daily calorie intake drops under 1,100, do not reduce calories further; speak to your physician.

Chapter 8

HEALTHY EATING: JANE'S DIET TIPS AND VARIETY MEAL PLANNER

*I*n nineteenth-century Nantucket, obesity was rare. The average person walked three to five miles per day. Most jobs required physical labor. My great-grandfather Captain John Conway worked his way up from cabin boy to crew member and eventually captain of a clipper ship that sailed around Cape Horn in the China trade. His job was at all times physically demanding. His diet consisted of fish, chowder, hardtack, salted beef, and a dram of rum. While not a balanced diet by today's standards, it supplied more than an adequate number of calories to sustain him in his shipboard activities. This was true for most of his contemporaries.

As decades passed, people became much more sedentary. Jobs became less physical. People rode or drove to work. Walking became an activity rather than a mode of transportation. At the same time, the amount and type of food consumed changed radically. Packaged and processed foods became the norm. Portion sizes dramatically increased. Fast foods became readily available. In the twentieth century, obesity was recognized as a public health problem. In the twenty-first century, it is seen as an epidemic.

Research has shown that Americans often underestimate the number of calories that they are consuming each day by as much as 25 percent.[1] This may be because most people incorrectly determine the appropriate portion sizes of the foods that they eat. Many individuals find it too difficult to remember lists of ounces, grams, cups, tablespoons, and the like. By using the Nantucket Diet Meal Planner, you should be able to gain an understanding of portion control. Measuring food amounts for several days will help you to begin to become familiar with the amounts that are in certain portions. For example, the more you measure a cup of cereal and place it in a bowl, spread a tablespoon of margarine on a piece of toast, or put a 3-ounce serving of chicken on a plate, the easier it will become for you to determine these measurements just by looking at them. Applying this knowledge will be an integral part of developing healthy eating habits.

A visualization technique may be an aid in correctly estimating portion size. Comparing serving amounts to familiar objects that you can visualize in your head or look at in front of you allows for making proper portion choices.[2] In addition to a calorie counter I have provided a portion chart on page 244 showing you some basic servings of foods and the approximate size of objects to which they compare.

THE NANTUCKET DIET MEAL PLANNING:
AS SIMPLE AS ABC

Poor eating habits lead to a vicious cycle of obesity, poor body image, and a sedentary lifestyle. The Nantucket Diet is a straightforward plan that allows you to gain control and break this cycle. Healthy eating begets a healthy lifestyle. It should not be perceived as onerous or necessarily restrictive. By embracing a healthy diet, you can live not only longer but also better. This is the ultimate message of our book.

Our variety meal planner is designed to give you a sample set of menus so that you can become familiar with the types of foods that you should be eating and the portion sizes. By no means do you need to follow this exact plan. If you feel comfortable enough using our calorie chart and following our recipes, you may create your own meal plan (as long as you stay within your calorie count). This is what we hope you will be able to ultimately accomplish. Remember, you are learning to change your lifestyle, not diet. Healthy meal planning will soon become second nature.

The daily meal plan includes a 1,200-calorie set menu for breakfast, lunch, dinner, and snacks. Everyone's plan will include all of the items that are on listed on the 1,200-calorie menu. You will then find a list of additions to the menu, divided into three categories (A, B, C). Each item listed as an A counts as 100 calories, each item listed as a B counts as 200 calories, and the items listed as a C count as 300 calories. You can choose whatever foods you would like from the "additions to menu" column to add to your menu, depending upon your calorie count. For instance, if during Phase 2 you consume 1,300 calories per day, you will eat everything that is on the 1,200-calorie menu plus one addition from the A list. If your Phase 2 calories are 1,600 per day, for example, you could choose two foods from the A list and one food from the B list, or one food from the A list and one food from the C list.

Other examples:

Calorie Level: 1,900

EAT	The 1,200-calorie menu plan for the day	+	2 A's (200 calories) 1 B (200 calories) 1 C (300 calories)	=	1,900

or

EAT	The 1,200-calorie menu plan for the day	+	4 A's (400 calories) 1 C (300 calories)	=	1,900

As long as you stay within your particular calorie count you can mix and match the daily set menus and the additions to the menu to create a multitude of menu options. For instance, you may select breakfast from plan 11, lunch from plan 6, and dinner and snacks from plan 7. If you look at breakfast, lunch, dinner, and snacks for each plan, you will see the calorie counts for all of the meals. You may mix and match them all you want as long as your daily total adds up to 1,200 calories for your set menu. Another option is to follow the set menus but choose additions to the menu from different days. For example, if you are following the set menu for plan 3, you can choose additions from plan 3 as well as additions to the menu from any of the other plans. The asterisks on the meal planner indicate recipes that are available in the book and can be found in the index. It is also possible to follow the meal planner but replace our suggested recipes with your own food selections if they contain the same number of calories. For example, you may wish to replace Family Favorite Meat Loaf with a piece of broiled chicken or even a low-calorie frozen dinner. Instead of preparing striped bass at home, you may prefer to go out to eat and have a piece of fish at a restaurant. It is important to realize that our variety meal planner is designed to be flexible so that it can easily become a part of your daily eating repertoire. Any one of the meals per week can be replaced by your Make Love to Life meal, which may consist of anything that you might be craving.

The Nantucket Diet Variety Meal Planner

PLAN 1

1,200-Calorie Menu

Breakfast: CALORIES 220

½ cup Kelloggs® All-Bran cereal with
Extra Fiber and ¾ cup skim milk,
topped with ½ cup fresh blueberries
½ grapefruit
Coffee with 2 tablespoons skim milk
Artificial sweetener to taste

Lunch: CALORIES 380

*Tuna Veggie Roll-Up
6 oz. fat-free yogurt
1 tangerine
Water or calorie-free flavored water

Dinner: CALORIES 380

*1 serving Whole-Grain Veggie
Lasagna
*1 Caesar Salad
2 tablespoons of calorie free or fat-free
dressing
Water or sparkling water

Snacks: CALORIES 220

4 cups popcorn, air-popped, no salt
3 apricots
*1 Mocha Frost

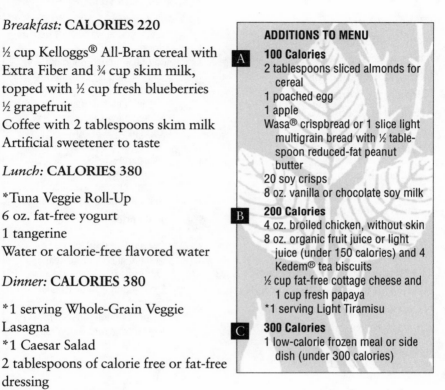

ADDITIONS TO MENU

A | **100 Calories**
2 tablespoons sliced almonds for cereal
1 poached egg
1 apple
Wasa® crispbread or 1 slice light multigrain bread with ½ tablespoon reduced-fat peanut butter
20 soy crisps
8 oz. vanilla or chocolate soy milk

B | **200 Calories**
4 oz. broiled chicken, without skin
8 oz. organic fruit juice or light juice (under 150 calories) and 4 Kedem® tea biscuits
½ cup fat-free cottage cheese and 1 cup fresh papaya
*1 serving Light Tiramisu

C | **300 Calories**
1 low-calorie frozen meal or side dish (under 300 calories)

GREAT PRODUCT CHOICES

Coffee: Nantucket Coffee Roasters Island Blend.
Salad dressing: Walden Farms® dressings are calorie-, carbohydrate-, and sugar-free.
Juice: Nantucket Nectars® Organic Banana Mango Carrot—100% Pure Organic Juice contains only 120 calories with 50 percent of the daily recommended allowance of vitamin C.
Soy crisps: The crunchy snack GeniSoy® is an alternative to chips without all the fat and calories and contains 7 grams of protein.
Tea Biscuits: Kedem ® biscuits are low in calories, sugar, and fat, and make a great snack.

PLAN 2

1,200-Calorie Menu

Breakfast: CALORIES 370

*Banana Oatmeal
½ cup nonfat cottage cheese
½ cup watermelon
1 cup light orange juice
Herb tea or coffee
Artificial sweetener to taste

Lunch: CALORIES 290

*Chicken Breast Sandwich
1 cup grapes
Sugar-free iced tea

Dinner: CALORIES 300

*1 serving Seared Nantucket Bay Scallops with Cranberry Papaya Salsa
*Nantucket Diet Wedge Salad
3.5 oz. wine of choice, preferably red

Snacks: CALORIES 240

1 protein or granola bar (140 calories or less)
1 Bosc pear
1 sugar-free popsicle

ADDITIONS TO MENU

A 100 Calories
2 tablespoons walnuts or pecans for oatmeal
Additional ½ cup nonfat cottage cheese and ½ cup watermelon
5 dried apricots
½ medium cantaloupe or 1½ cups cubed pieces
1 cup steamed asparagus, 1 tablespoon squeezable nonfat margarine. NoSalt® (salt substitute), pepper, and ½ cup tomatoes with 1 tablespoon parmesan cheese for salad

B 200 Calories
15 veggie chips
*1 serving of Kale Soup
1 additional serving of scallops with salsa
*1 serving of Nantucket Diet Fake Fries
*1 Light Cannoli (dessert)
*1 Blueberry Tofu Smoothie

GREAT PRODUCT CHOICES
Wine: Nantucket Vineyards Dry Pinot Noir is a full-flavored, smooth wine that is a perfect accompaniment to light dishes.
Protein bar: Biochem® Ultimate Protein Bar™, Chocolate Chocolate Dream, has 140 calories, 15 grams of protein, 6 grams of sugar, and 2.5 grams of fat; Diabetitrim®, Peanut Butter, has 130 calories, 10 grams of protein, 1 gram of sugar, 3.5 grams of fat, and 4 grams of fiber.
Granola bar: Nature Valley® trail mix bars, Quaker® Q-Smart snack bars.
Veggie chips: Robert's American Gourmet®, a healthy, all-natural snack.

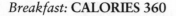

PLAN 3

1,200-Calorie Menu

Breakfast: **CALORIES 360**

1 whole-wheat English muffin
1 tablespoon margarine (Benecol®
Light)
2 tablespoons sugar-free strawberry
jam
1 cup chocolate soy milk
2 kiwi fruits
Coffee with 2 tablespoons skim milk
Artificial sweetener to taste

Lunch: **CALORIES 260**

*1 Tropical Fruit Salad with Pineapple
Vinaigrette
1 (28 g) mini whole wheat pita bread
Water or diet soda

Dinner: **CALORIES 340**

*1 serving Family Favorite Meat Loaf
1 cup steamed broccoli with 2 teaspoons imitation cheese sprinkles
*1 serving Sweet Winter Squash
Water or calorie-free flavored water

Snacks: **CALORIES 240**

*1 Chocolate Protein Shake
*4 cups Sweet Cinnamon Popcorn

> **ADDITIONS TO MENU**
>
> **A** **100 Calories**
> Replace margarine with 1 table-
> spoon reduced-fat peanut but-
> ter
> 1 Wasa® crispbread with 1 slice
> fat-free cheddar cheese (place
> in microwave for 10 seconds to
> melt cheese, if desired)
> 6 oz. yogurt
> 5 dried prunes
>
> **B** **200 Calories**
> 8 oz. organic juice or light juice
> (under 150 calories) and 1 cup
> watermelon
> 1 cup wheat flakes cereal with ½
> cup skim milk and artificial
> sweetener
> 1 cup cooked long-grain brown
> rice
> ¼ cup dry roasted mixed nuts
> *1 serving Nantucket Blueberry
> Shortcake
> 1 additional serving meatloaf

GREAT PRODUCT CHOICES

Margarine: *Benecol®, Take Control,* and *Smart Balance®* all contain zero trans fats and may
help to lower cholesterol.

Soy milk: *Soy Slender*™ is great-tasting and has only 70 calories per cup.

Juice: *Nantucket Nectars®* Organic Cloudy Apple—100% Pure Organic Juice contains only
120 calories and has 100 percent of the recommended daily allowance of vitamin C.

PLAN 4

1,200-Calorie Menu

Breakfast: **CALORIES 290**

1 poached egg
*1 Mixed Berry Muffin
Coffee with 2 tablespoons skim milk
Artificial sweetener to taste

Lunch: **CALORIES 285**

*Ham and Pickle Pita
Water or calorie-free flavored water

Dinner: **CALORIES 520**

*1 Serving Sfoglia Mussels
*1 serving Whole-Wheat Spaghetti
with Lemon, Almond, and Dandelion
Greens
3 cups mixed green salad
2 tablespoons calorie free dressing
Sugar-free iced tea

Snacks: **CALORIES 105**

1 apple
1 sugar-free popsicle

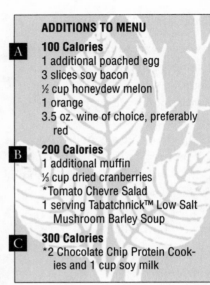

ADDITIONS TO MENU

A 100 Calories
1 additional poached egg
3 slices soy bacon
½ cup honeydew melon
1 orange
3.5 oz. wine of choice, preferably
  red

B 200 Calories
1 additional muffin
⅓ cup dried cranberries
*Tomato Chevre Salad
1 serving Tabatchnick™ Low Salt
  Mushroom Barley Soup

C 300 Calories
*2 Chocolate Chip Protein Cook-
  ies and 1 cup soy milk

GREAT PRODUCT CHOICES
Coffee: Nantucket Coffee Roasters Sconset Blend.
Wine: Nantucket Vineyards Merlot is a deep, earthy red wine.

PLAN 5

1,200-Calorie Menu

Breakfast: **CALORIES 250**

1 cup toasted oat cereal and
1 cup skim milk topped with
½ cup raspberries
Tea with 2 tablespoons skim milk
Artificial sweetener to taste

Lunch: **CALORIES 415**

*1 serving Chicken Soup
3 cups mixed green salad
2 tablespoons fat-free dressing
½ grapefruit
Water or sparkling water

Dinner: **CALORIES 345**

*1 serving Ham with Pineapple
*1 Spinach Salad with Dijon Dressing
Water or calorie-free flavored water

Snacks: **CALORIES 190**

4 oz. unsweetened applesauce
¼ cup soy nuts

ADDITIONS TO MENU

A **100 Calories**
6 oz. yogurt
10 Wheat Thins® low-salt
   crackers
1 cup cherries
*3 Chocolate-Dipped Strawber-
   ries

B **200 Calories**
*1 Veggie Pocket Sandwich
1 additional serving of Ham with
   Pineapple
*1 serving Green Beans Alman-
   dine
8 oz. organic juice or light juice
   (under 150 calories) and
   2 Joseph's® bite size sugar-free
   cookies.

C **300 Calories**
*3 Chocolate Almond Cookies
   with 1 cup skim milk
*1 Tropical Tofu Shake

GREAT PRODUCT CHOICES

Juice: Nantucket Nectars® Organic Blueberry Banana.
Cookies: Joseph's® bite size sugar-free cookies come in a variety of flavors, have only 100 calories in 4 cookies and are a perfect way to satisfy a sweet craving.

PLAN 6

1,200-Calorie Menu

Breakfast: **CALORIES 280**

*Fluffy Veggie Omelet for One
2-inch slice of melon
8 oz. vanilla almond soy milk

Lunch: **CALORIES 300**

Nantucket Diet Dog: 1 turkey, soy, or
chicken hot dog (low sodium) in 1 light
whole-wheat hot dog bun with 1 tablespoon ketchup, 1 tablespoon relish, 1
teaspoon mustard, and 1 tablespoon
chopped onion
3 cups mixed green salad
2 tablespoons fat-free dressing
Iced coffee with 2 tablespoons skim
milk and artificial sweetener to taste

Dinner: **CALORIES 400**

*1 serving Tuckernuck Inn Café
Paper Bag Catch
2 cups salad with calorie-free dressing
Water or diet soda

Snacks: **CALORIES 220**

½ sliced banana and ¼ cup fresh blueberries
20 soy crisps
1 nectarine

ADDITIONS TO MENU

A 100 Calories
1 cup puffed rice cereal with ½
cup skim milk and artificial
sweetener to taste
½ cup fat-free plain yogurt with ½
cup fresh blackberries
1 cup fresh broccoli and 1 cup
fresh cauliflower with 2 tablespoons fat-free dip
10 low-salt, low-fat pretzels
3.5 oz. wine of choice, preferably
red

B 200 Calories
1 graham cracker (4 sections),
original or chocolate with
1 tablespoon reduced-fat
peanut butter
1 additional turkey, soy, or
chicken dog, bun, and condi-
ments
1 cup fat-free, sugar-free ice
cream or frozen yogurt
½ additional serving Tuckernuck
Inn Café Paper Bag Catch

C 300 Calories
*1 serving Pumpkin Maple Pie

GREAT PRODUCT CHOICES
Dip: Marzetti's® fat-free dips are low in calories and add lots of flavor to raw vegetables.
Wine: Nantucket Vineyards Prodeano is a light Prosecco-style wine perfect for a premeal toast
or great for a beach picnic.

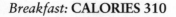

PLAN 7

1,200-Calorie Menu

Breakfast: CALORIES 310

2 fat-free frozen waffles
2 tablespoons sugar-free maple syrup
1 cup blueberries and ½ cup strawberries in ½ cup skim milk
Herb tea with 2 tablespoons skim milk
Artificial sweetener to taste

Lunch: CALORIES 300

*1 Apple Tofu Salad with Raspberry Lime Vinaigrette
Water or sparkling water

Dinner: CALORIES 290

*1 slice Whole-Wheat Cheese Pizza
3 cups mixed green salad
2 tablespoons fat-free dressing

Snacks: CALORIES 300

15 soy tortilla chips with ½ cup salsa
1 fat-free ice cream sandwich

ADDITIONS TO MENU

A **100 Calories**
1 whole grapefruit
2 caramel rice cakes
6 oz. yogurt
1 light beer

B **200 Calories**
5 slices melba toast with 2 tablespoons low-fat cream cheese and ¼ cup slices of banana
5 medium dates
*1 Banana Strawberry Fruit Smoothie
*1 serving Pineapple Upside-Down Cake

C **300 Calories**
1 additional slice of pizza
*BLT Light Sandwich

GREAT PRODUCT CHOICES

Maple syrup: *Howard's®* sugar-free syrup has only 2 calories in a ¼ cup serving, 1 gram of carbohydrate, and 0 grams of fat and sugar.

Tortilla chips: *Keto™ Chips* are a healthy snack with 12 grams of protein and 4 grams of fiber per serving.

PLAN 8

1,200-Calorie Menu

Breakfast: **CALORIES 220**

1½ cups puffed wheat cereal and ½ cup
skim milk
½ cup nonfat cottage cheese with ⅓ cup
sliced banana
Coffee with 2 tablespoons skim milk
Artificial sweetener to taste

Lunch: **CALORIES 340**

*1 Lobster Roll
3 cups mixed green salad
2 tablespoons calorie-free dressing
1 apple
Water or diet soda

Dinner: **CALORIES 360**

*1 serving Veal Marsala
1 cup steamed Brussels sprouts
1 cup steamed beets
1 tablespoon squeezable nonfat margarine and seasoning to taste
Water or sparkling water

Snacks: **CALORIES 280**

*1 Chicken Taco
2 plums

ADDITIONS TO MENU

A **100 Calories**
1 slice light whole-wheat toast
with ½ tablespoon Benecol®
Light and 1 tablespoon sugar-
free grape jelly
5 cups popcorn, air-popped, no
salt
1 serving Tabatchnick™ Cabbage
Soup
3.5 oz. wine of choice, preferably
red

B **200 Calories**
*1 Nantucket Diet Bran Muffin
*1 serving Cinnamon Toast
½ additional serving Veal Marsala
Sushi, 4 pieces
*1 prepared protein drink (under
200 calories)

C **300 Calories**
*1 Sugar-Free Rocky Road Ice
Cream Sandwich

GREAT PRODUCT CHOICES
Margarine: Smart Beat®, Smart Squeeze has zero trans fatty acids and only 5 calories per
tablespoon.
Soup: Tabatchnick™ frozen soups have varieties that are low-calorie, low-sodium, and high in
fiber. They are a healthy, filling food choice.
Wine: Nantucket Vineyards Syrah has a wonderful berry flavor, perfect for meats and heavier
dishes.

PLAN 9

1,200-Calorie Menu

Breakfast: **CALORIES 350**

*Apple Cinnamon Oatmeal
½ cup fat-free yogurt
1 sliced peach
1 cup light grapefruit juice

Lunch: **CALORIES 400**

*1 serving Cream of Broccoli Soup
*1 Chicken Caesar Salad
Iced coffee with 2 tablespoons skim
milk and artificial sweetener to taste

Dinner: **CALORIES 300**

*1 serving Indian Roasted Pork Loin
with Zesty Marinade
2 cups steamed broccoli and cauliflower with seasoning to taste

Snacks: **CALORIES 150**

2 kiwi fruits
1 sugar-free Creamsicle

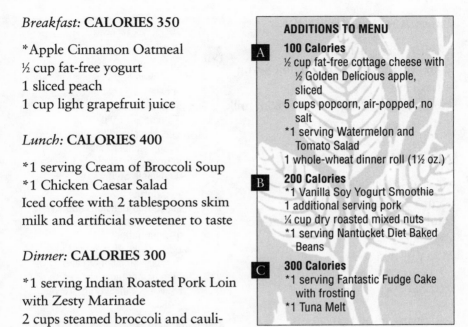

ADDITIONS TO MENU

A 100 Calories
½ cup fat-free cottage cheese with
   ½ Golden Delicious apple,
   sliced
5 cups popcorn, air-popped, no
   salt
*1 serving Watermelon and
   Tomato Salad
1 whole-wheat dinner roll (1½ oz.)

B 200 Calories
*1 Vanilla Soy Yogurt Smoothie
1 additional serving pork
¼ cup dry roasted mixed nuts
*1 serving Nantucket Diet Baked
   Beans

C 300 Calories
*1 serving Fantastic Fudge Cake
   with frosting
*1 Tuna Melt

GREAT PRODUCT CHOICES

Chicken: Purdue® low-fat breaded chicken breasts are easy to prepare and are only 140 calories.

PLAN 10

1,200-Calorie Menu

Breakfast: **CALORIES 240**

*2 slices French Toast
2 tablespoons sugar-free maple syrup
4 fresh apricots
Herb tea with 2 tablespoons skim milk
Artificial sweetener to taste

Lunch: **CALORIES 250**

*Terrific Turkey Wrap
3 cups mixed green salad
2 tablespoons calorie-free or fat-free
dressing
Water or diet soda

Dinner: **CALORIES 440**

*1 serving Fisherman's Feast
1 cup wax beans, seasoned to taste
1 cup steamed spinach
*1 Chocolate Soy Yogurt Smoothie

Snacks: **CALORIES 270**

¼ cup dry roasted peanuts
1 Bartlett pear

ADDITIONS TO MENU

A   100 Calories
3 slices low-fat bacon
*4 carrot sticks 4 inches long and
    4 celery sticks 4 inches long
    with 3 tablespoons *Zesty
    Tomato Tofu Dip
½ cup nonfat cottage cheese and
    ½ cup blueberries
1 serving Tabatchnick™ Low Salt
    Vegetable Soup

B   200 Calories
1 sliced Red Delicious apple with
    1 tablespoon reduced-fat
    peanut butter
8 oz. organic juice or light juice
    (under 150 calories) and
    8 mini meringue cookies
*1 serving Vanilla Chip Brownie
    Cake

C   300 Calories
1 cup cooked whole-wheat pasta
    with 2 tablespoons parmesan
    cheese
1 low-calorie frozen meal or side
    dish (under 300 calories)

GREAT PRODUCT CHOICES
Juice: Nantucket Nectars® Organic Very Raspberry.
Meringue cookies: Bakehouse Foods Inc. Gourmet mini cookies are fat-free and contain
approximately 7 calories per piece.

PLAN 11

1,200-Calorie Menu

Breakfast: **CALORIES 300**

Omelet made with ¾ cup egg substitute, ¼ cup tomatoes, and ¼ cup mushrooms, prepared using nonstick cooking spray
1 slice light whole-wheat toast
½ tablespoon Benecol® Light
1 tablespoon sugar-free raspberry jam
1 tangerine
Coffee with 2 tablespoons skim milk
Artificial sweetener to taste

Lunch: **CALORIES 250**

* 1 Shrimp Salad with Tomato Vinaigrette
1 cup fresh pineapple
Sugar-free iced tea

Dinner: **CALORIES 450**

3 oz. lean grilled steak
*Grilled Onions and Peppers
2 tablespoons A-1® steak sauce
*1 serving Glazed Carrots
*1 serving Cauliflower Italienne

Snacks: **CALORIES 200**

2 sugar-free fudgesicles
1 banana

ADDITIONS TO MENU

A 100 Calories
1 cup fresh mixed berries
1 slice light whole-wheat toast with ½ tablespoon Benecol® Light and 1 tablespoon sugar-free raspberry jam
1 nectarine
1 sugar-free ice cream bar (100 calories or less)
1 3.5 oz. wine of choice, preferably red

B 200 Calories
*Vanilla Oatmeal
*4 cups Cheese Popcorn
*1 Veggie Pita Pizza

C 300 Calories
Additional 3 oz. serving of steak
*1 serving Quick Key Lime Pie

GREAT PRODUCT CHOICES

Iced tea: Nantucket Nectars® Squeezed Diet Lemon Tea has zero calories and 100 percent of the recommended allowance of vitamin C.
Wine: Nantucket Vineyards Sailors Delight, a blend of Pinot Noir, Merlot, Chardonnay, and Syrah, is a full-bodied wine that's a great accompaniment to meats and is perfect for barbecues.

PLAN 12

1,200-Calorie Menu

Breakfast: **CALORIES 260**

*1 serving Whole-Wheat Pancakes
2 tablespoons sugar-free maple syrup
½ grapefruit
1 cup light orange juice

Lunch: **CALORIES 410**

Nantucket Diet Burger: 1 veggie burger
patty, 1 light whole-wheat burger bun,
1 tablespoon ketchup, 1 tablespoon
mustard, 2 lettuce leaves, 2 tomato
slices, 1 onion slice
*1 Cranberry Walnut Salad with
Cranberry Dressing
Iced coffee with artificial sweetener

Dinner: **CALORIES 320**

*1 serving Crispy Chicken Dijon
1 steamed ear of corn, squeezable nonfat margarine, NoSalt® (salt substitute)
and pepper to taste
1 cup steamed spinach, seasoned to
taste
Water or calorie-free flavored water

Snacks: **CALORIES 210**

1 protein or granola bar (140 calories or less)
*1 Chocolate Frost

ADDITIONS TO MENU

A 100 Calories
½ cup Kellogg's® All-Bran cereal
with Extra Fiber, ¾ cup skim
milk, artificial sweetener to
taste
*1 serving of Nantucket Diet Fried
Cinnamon Apples (great for
pancakes)
½ cup sugar-free chocolate or pistachio pudding prepared using
instant mix, 2 tablespoons fat-
free imitation whipped topping
Additional veggie burger patty, no
bun
2 tangerines
1 D'Anjou pear
1 additional ear of corn

B 200 Calories
4 melba toasts with 2 tablespoons
low-fat cream cheese and ¼
cup strawberry slices
1 banana, sliced and topped with
2 tablespoons sugar-free
chocolate syrup and 2 tablespoons fat-free imitation
whipped topping
1 additional serving Crispy
Chicken Dijon

GREAT PRODUCT CHOICES
Seasoning: *Mrs. Dash® Seasonings* are calorie- and salt-free and add great flavor to foods.
Syrup: Sweet 'n Low flavored syrups are sugar-free, fat-free and contain only 15 calories in
2 tablespoons.
Tip: Choose protein bars high in protein and fiber, low in sugar and calories.

PLAN 13

1,200-Calorie Menu

Breakfast: **CALORIES 260**

1 multigrain bagel
2 tablespoons fat-free cream cheese
1 peach
1 cup skim milk

Lunch: **CALORIES 400**

*1 serving Chicken Paprikash
*1 Mandarin Salad
Water or diet soda

Dinner: **CALORIES 400**

*Paillards of Striped Bass Sautéed with
Mesclun Greens and Virgin Tomato
Sauce
1½ cups steamed green beans
1 cup steamed summer squash with 1
tablespoon squeezable nonfat mar-
garine, NoSalt® or Salt Sense® (salt substitute), and pepper to taste
Water

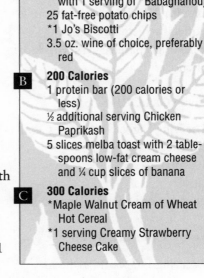

ADDITIONS TO MENU

A **100 Calories**
6 oz. yogurt
*1 cup red and green peppers
   with 1 serving of *Babaghanouj
25 fat-free potato chips
*1 Jo's Biscotti
3.5 oz. wine of choice, preferably
   red

B **200 Calories**
1 protein bar (200 calories or
   less)
½ additional serving Chicken
   Paprikash
5 slices melba toast with 2 tablespoons low-fat cream cheese
   and ¼ cup slices of banana

C **300 Calories**
*Maple Walnut Cream of Wheat
   Hot Cereal
*1 serving Creamy Strawberry
   Cheese Cake

Snacks: **CALORIES 140**

1 cup green grapes
*1 Coffee Frost

GREAT PRODUCT CHOICES

Protein bar: *Kashi* ® *Go Lean* Crunch Peanut Bliss contains 170 calories, 9 grams of protein, and 5 grams of fiber—a filling snack. *Power Bar* ® *Sugar Free Protein Plus* contains 170 calories, 16 grams of protein, and 0 grams of sugar.

Wine: *Nantucket Vineyards* Pinot Gris has melon and strawberry notes and an earthy, long-lasting finish. Great for seafood and lighter dishes.

Salt: NoSalt® and NuSalt®, for those of you on salt-restricted diets. These substitutes have the flavor of real salt without the sodium (contains potassium). Salt Sense®, for those of you sensitive to potassium, this substitute has 33% less sodium per serving than real salt.

PLAN 14

1,200-Calorie Menu

Breakfast: **CALORIES 300**

1 cup bran flakes cereal with 1 small
box raisins and 1 cup skim milk
1 cup watermelon
Tea with 2 tablespoons skim milk
Artificial sweetener to taste or
1 packet prepared Swiss Miss® diet
hot chocolate

Lunch: **CALORIES 350**

*1 serving Light Nantucket Clam
Chowder
*1 Crab Cake
1 apple
Water or zero-calorie flavored water

Dinner: **CALORIES 320**

*1 serving Eggplant Parmesan
*1 Greek Salad

Snacks: **CALORIES 230**

4 oz. sugar-free Jell-O® with 3 tablespoons fat-free imitation whipped
topping
1 rice cake with 1 slice fat-free cheese
1 cup cherries

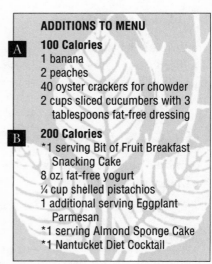

ADDITIONS TO MENU

A **100 Calories**
1 banana
2 peaches
40 oyster crackers for chowder
2 cups sliced cucumbers with 3
   tablespoons fat-free dressing

B **200 Calories**
*1 serving Bit of Fruit Breakfast
   Snacking Cake
8 oz. fat-free yogurt
¼ cup shelled pistachios
1 additional serving Eggplant
   Parmesan
*1 serving Almond Sponge Cake
*1 Nantucket Diet Cocktail

GREAT PRODUCT CHOICES
Hot chocolate: *Swiss Miss*® Diet contains only 25 calories and has as much calcium as an
8 oz. glass of milk.

Chapter 9

NANTUCKET'S BEST RECIPES

*O*ur recipe section includes over one hundred low-calorie, nutritious, and delicious dishes. You will find a section titled "Nantucket Old-Time Family Favorites" with some of the island's most popular recipes, some dating back a century. "Dining Out" contains delectable recipe choices from many of the island's top restaurants and cafés along with dining tips to help guide you toward lower-calorie options when you eat out. The "Special Events" section includes low-calorie recipes from Nantucket's top caterers. It also features a party segment, highlighting clambakes, luncheons, and the "thrill of the grill." "Simple Pleasures" is designed for those of you who do not have the time to cook or the desire to do so but want to make healthy food choices—we have selected several quick and easy low-calorie meals and snacks that will satisfy your needs. "Holiday Cheer" gives you alternatives to traditional holiday favorites. Recipes that are designated as "Make Love to Life" are fantastic choices for the one meal a week that you do not strictly adhere to the guidelines of the diet. Finally, you will find a section called "Off-

Island Gourmet" with a delectable collection of low-calorie recipes from two of New York and Boston's finest restaurants.

All of the recipes include a full nutritional analysis, and many are perfect for diabetics and vegetarians. Not only are the recipes we have compiled healthy dining options, but we think they will please even the most discerning palate.

Our recipes have letters from A to J next to them indicating the number of calories per serving in each recipe. This will make it simpler for you to calculate your daily calorie intake. For example, a recipe with a calorie count of 580 would be an F; one with 60 calories would be an A. As indicated in our Meal Planner instructions, when you count your daily calories, the additions to the menu and recipes must be counted at the higher calorie number. For example, a B is counted at 200; a G is counted at 700; and so on.

It is much more beneficial to overestimate the number of calories that you are consuming. This method allows for any portion issues—for instance, if you eat a larger serving than you should for one of your meals, or if you choose a large banana as opposed to a small banana. By using our calorie counting method, even if your final calorie count turns out to be lower than it should, the only thing that will result is a faster weight loss. This is a good thing.

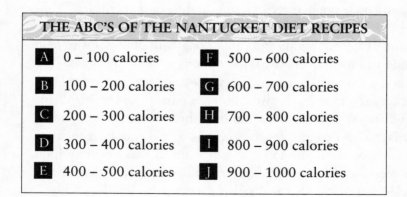

THE ABC'S OF THE NANTUCKET DIET RECIPES		
A	0 – 100 calories	F	500 – 600 calories
B	100 – 200 calories	G	600 – 700 calories
C	200 – 300 calories	H	700 – 800 calories
D	300 – 400 calories	I	800 – 900 calories
E	400 – 500 calories	J	900 – 1000 calories

Nantucket Old-Time Family Favorites

This section contains favorite Nantucket recipes. Some of them have been updated to adhere to the low-calorie guidelines of the Nantucket Diet.

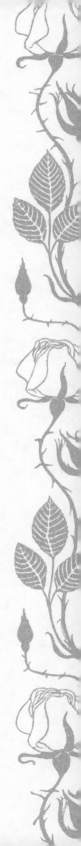

BREAKFAST

Bit of Fruit Breakfast Snacking Cake

Serves: 12

2½ cups all-purpose flour
¼ cup light brown sugar, packed
4 tablespoons margarine (Benecol® or
    similar)
1 16-oz. can no-sugar-added or light
    fruit cocktail (reserve ⅓ cup juice)
½ cup egg substitute
1 teaspoon vanilla extract
2 teaspoons baking soda
½ teaspoon NoSalt® (salt substitute)
Nonstick butter-flavored cooking
    spray

Mix all ingredients together except the fruit. Beat on medium for three minutes. Add the fruit using a spoon so as not to crush the fruit. Spray a 13-by-9-inch pan with butter-flavored spray. Pour mixture into pan. Bake at 350 degrees for 20 to 25 minutes or until a toothpick comes out clean.

NUTRITIONAL ANALYSIS PER SERVING	Calories	194	Fiber	1 g
	Carbohydrates	29 g	Protein	4 g
	Sugar	9 g	Calcium	18 mg
	Total Fat	6.6 g	Vitamin A	491 I.U.
	Saturated Fat	0.8 g	Vitamin C	1 mg
	Cholesterol	0 mg	Folate	50 mcg
	Sodium	306 mg		

Nantucket Diet Bran Muffins

B   *Serves:* 8

1 cup Kellogg's® All-Bran Cereal with
    Extra Fiber
1 cup skim milk
¾ cup Splenda®
1 egg
¼ cup vegetable oil
1 cup whole-wheat flour
2 teaspoons baking powder
¼ teaspoon NoSalt® (salt substitute)
Nonstick cooking spray
2 tablespoons Splenda® for topping

Place cereal and milk in large bowl. Let sit for 3 minutes. Mix in all remaining ingredients. Coat 8 muffin pan cups with nonstick cooking spray. Fill each cup about two-thirds full. Bake at 400 degrees for 15 to 20 minutes. When cool, remove from pan. Place on plate. Sprinkle with Splenda®.

NUTRITIONAL ANALYSIS PER SERVING				
Calories	156	Fiber	6 g
Carbohydrates	21 g	Protein	5 g
Sugar	0 g	Calcium	136 mg
Total Fat	8.2 g	Vitamin A	248 I.U.
Saturated Fat	0.8 g	Vitamin C	2 mg
Cholesterol	27 mg	Folate	43 mcg
Sodium	181 mg		

Mixed Berry Muffins

Serves: 8

1½ cups all-purpose flour
¼ cup sugar
¼ cup plus 2 tablespoons Splenda®
    (sugar substitute)
½ teaspoon NoSalt® (salt substitute)
1 egg
¼ cup vegetable oil or corn oil
½ cup skim milk
2 teaspoons baking powder
1 cup frozen mixed berries
Nonstick cooking spray

Combine all ingredients except berries. Fold berries into mixture. Coat 8 muffin pan cups with nonstick cooking spray. Fill cups two-thirds full with batter. Bake at 375 degrees for 15 to 20 minutes.

NUTRITIONAL ANALYSIS PER SERVING				
	Calories	199	Fiber	1 g
	Carbohydrates	29 g	Protein	4 g
	Sugar	8 g	Calcium	94 mg
	Total Fat	7.9 g	Vitamin A	76 I.U.
	Saturated Fat	0.7 g	Vitamin C	0 mg
	Cholesterol	27 mg	Folate	53 mcg
	Sodium	138 mg		

Whole-Wheat Pancakes

Serves: 5

1 cup whole-wheat flour
1 tablespoon sugar
2 tablespoons Splenda®
¼ teaspoon NoSalt® (salt substitute)
2 teaspoons baking powder
½ cup skim milk
2 eggs
1 teaspoon corn oil
Nonstick cooking spray
Sugar-free maple syrup or fresh fruit
    (for topping)

In a mixing bowl combine all ingredients. Coat a frying pan well with nonstick cooking spray. For each pancake, place about ⅓ cup of batter into pan. Cook over medium heat until golden on each side. Serve with sugar-free maple syrup or top with fresh fruit.

NUTRITIONAL ANALYSIS PER SERVING				
Calories	140	Fiber	3 g
Carbohydrates	22 g	Protein	7 g
Sugar	3 g	Calcium	151 mg
Total Fat	3.4 g	Vitamin A	150 I.U.
Saturated Fat	0.8 g	Vitamin C	0 mg
Cholesterol	85 mg	Folate	21 mcg
Sodium	235 mg		

LUNCH

Tropical Fruit Salad with Pineapple Vinaigrette

Serves: 1

2–3 cups chopped lettuce
¼ cup fat-free cottage cheese
⅓ cup diced fresh pineapple
½ cup diced fresh papaya
⅓ cup diced fresh mango
½ banana, sliced
2½ tablespoons shredded coconut
2 tablespoons Pineapple Vinaigrette
    (recipe follows)

Place lettuce in a large salad bowl. Top with cottage cheese, fruit, and vinaigrette. Sprinkle coconut on top.

NUTRITIONAL ANALYSIS PER SERVING				
	Calories	264	Fiber	4 g
	Carbohydrates	48 g	Protein	9 g
	Sugar	28 g	Calcium	93 mg
	Total Fat	5.8 g	Vitamin A	1,828 I.U.
	Saturated Fat	4.7 g	Vitamin C	60 mg
	Cholesterol	3 mg	Folate	102 mcg
	Sodium	271 mg		

Pineapple Vinaigrette

Serves: 6 (2 tablespoons per serving)

6 ounces pineapple juice
1 tablespoon red wine vinegar
½ tablespoon cornstarch
2 packages Equal®

Place pineapple juice, vinegar, and cornstarch in a microwave-safe bowl. Mix well. Heat for 2 minutes, until it comes to a boil. Stir (should be thickened like a salad dressing). Mix in artificial sweetener and place in refrigerator until nice and cold (1 hour).

NUTRITIONAL ANALYSIS PER SERVING					
Calories	13		Fiber	0 g
Carbohydrates	3 g		Protein	0 g
Sugar	2 g		Calcium	3 mg
Total Fat	0 g		Vitamin A	1 I.U.
Saturated Fat	0 g		Vitamin C	2 mg
Cholesterol	0 mg		Folate	4 mcg
Sodium	0 mg			

Nantucket Light Clam Chowder

Serves: 6

2 slices reduced-fat bacon
½ cup finely chopped onion
¼ cup finely chopped celery
2 garlic cloves, peeled and crushed
2 cups low-sodium chicken broth
3 tablespoons flour

½ cup potatoes, diced
1 10-ounce can whole baby clams
2 cups reduced-fat (2%) milk
Nonstick cooking spray

Place bacon in skillet. Cook until crisp. Set aside. Spray skillet with non-stick cooking spray. Add onion and celery. Cook until tender. (Do not brown.) Add garlic; mix and set aside. Place chicken broth in saucepan, but save 3–4 tablespoons and mix it with the flour. Let broth come to a boil and add broth and flour mixture. Continue to boil and stir until liquid is smooth and begins to thicken. Add potato and simmer until tender. Stir in onion, celery, and garlic. Add clams and milk. Simmer for 5–10 minutes. Garnish with crumbled bacon.

NUTRITIONAL ANALYSIS PER SERVING				
Calories	142	Fiber	1 g
Carbohydrates	14 g	Protein	13 g
Sugar	6 g	Calcium	185 mg
Total Fat	4.4 g	Vitamin A	381 I.U.
Saturated Fat	2 g	Vitamin C	4 mg
Cholesterol	47 mg	Folate	17 mcg
Sodium	377 mg		

Cream of Broccoli Soup

Serves: 10

1½ pounds broccoli
5 cups low-sodium chicken broth
2 tablespoons margarine (Benecol® or similar)
1 chopped onion
3 celery stalks, minced
¼ cup flour
2 cups reduced-fat (2%) milk

¼ teaspoon nutmeg
Salt to taste (optional)
Paprika to taste
Grated parmesan (1 tablespoon per
    bowl)

Wash broccoli, cut off florets, and set them aside. Peel stems and chop coarsely. Place stems and broth in large saucepan. Bring to boil and simmer 30 minutes. Drain, reserving liquid. Put the stems in a blender with 1 cup reserved liquid and blend. Set puree aside. Put florets in remaining liquid, bring to boil, simmer 5–7 minutes. Melt margarine in saucepan, sauté onion and celery for 5 minutes. Stir in flour and cook 3–4 minutes. Slowly stir in florets and liquid and bring to boil. Add puree and milk. Bring to boil. Add nutmeg, salt, and paprika to taste. Remove from heat. Serve with cheese.

NUTRITIONAL ANALYSIS PER SERVING	Calories	93	Fiber	1.4 g
	Carbohydrates	10 g	Protein	6 g
	Sugar	2 g	Calcium	144 mg
	Total Fat	3 g	Vitamin A	443 I.U.
	Saturated Fat	1.7 g	Vitamin C	39 mg
	Cholesterol	9.8 mg	Folate	42 mcg
	Sodium	166 mg		

Frances's Kale Soup

A traditional Portuguese soup. This family recipe has been updated to lower the calorie and fat content. We have also included the original because it is so typically Nantucket.

Serves: 10

1 cup dried red beans
1 pound chicken, white, skinless,
    boneless, cut into 1-inch cubes
1 pound kale, washed and torn into
    pieces
2 tablespoons margarine (Benecol®) or
    similar
1 medium onion, chopped
2 cups cubed potatoes
10 cups water
Salt and pepper to taste

Soak beans overnight in cold water. In the morning drain beans and put in a pot with chicken (cut chicken into pieces before placing in pot), kale, salt, and pepper. Fry onion in margarine and add to pot. Add 10 cups of water and bring to a boil, then reduce heat and simmer 2 to 3 hours. Add potatoes and 1 more cup of water. Cook until potatoes are tender.

(The original recipe is made with 1 pound of linguica sausage instead of chicken and ¼ pound of salt pork is added as well. You can try this on a Make Love to Life day. The traditional dish has 336 calories per serving.)

NUTRITIONAL ANALYSIS PER SERVING				
	Calories	175	Fiber	4 g
	Carbohydrates	21 g	Protein	11 g
	Sugar	2 g	Calcium	63 mg
	Total Fat	5.6 g	Vitamin A	4,298 I.U.
	Saturated Fat	1.5 g	Vitamin C	41 mg
	Cholesterol	24 mg	Folate	87 mcg
	Sodium	39 mg		

Chicken Paprikash

 Serves: 6

6 skinless, boneless chicken breasts
    (about 3 ounces each)
4 tablespoons margarine
1 teaspoon vegetable oil
2 cups diced onion
1 garlic clove, mashed (optional)
2 tablespoons paprika
1 tablespoon NoSalt® (salt substitute)
Pepper to taste
1 cup low-salt chicken broth
1 cup light or fat-free sour cream
1½ tablespoons cornstarch
Parsley for garnish
(optional) Whole-wheat cooked pasta
    for serving, 1 cup (not included in
    analysis) adds 175 calories

Melt margarine in large skillet. Cook chicken breasts on both sides until golden brown. Cut into chunks and put aside. Cook onions and garlic in oil until browned. Remove from heat and add paprika, NoSalt®, and pepper to taste. Stir well, add chicken broth, and bring to a boil. Reduce heat to low. Add chicken to mixture and cook 15–20 minutes. Combine cornstarch and sour cream. Stir well. Add slowly to pan, stirring well over very low heat until mixture is thickened. Garnish with parsley. Serve with whole-wheat pasta.

NUTRITIONAL ANALYSIS PER SERVING				
	Calories	243	Fiber	2 g
	Carbohydrates	14 g	Protein	22 g
	Sugar	5 g	Calcium	95 mg
	Total Fat	11 g	Vitamin A	1,726 I.U.
	Saturated Fat	3 g	Vitamin C	6 mg
	Cholesterol	63 mg	Folate	16 mcg
	Sodium	189 mg		

DINNER AND SIDE DISHES

Whole-Wheat Cheese Pizza

 Serves: 8

1 packet active dry yeast
1 cup warm water
1 teaspoon NoSalt® (salt substitute)
3 tablespoons olive oil
2½ cups whole-wheat flour
1½ cups Ragú® light chunky prima-
    vera tomato sauce
1 cup low-fat shredded mozzarella
Nonstick cooking spray

In a large bowl dissolve yeast in warm water. Add in NoSalt®, olive oil, and flour. Knead dough until smooth. Roll dough out onto floured wax paper. Let dough rise for about one hour. Mold into round 12-inch pizza pan well coated with nonstick cooking spray. Spread tomato sauce over dough and sprinkle with cheese. Bake at 450 degrees for 10–15 minutes. *Variation:* Top dough and sauce with your favorite fresh vegetables, mushrooms, peppers, etc., and then sprinkle with cheese and bake.

NUTRITIONAL ANALYSIS PER SERVING				
	Calories	221	Fiber	6 g
	Carbohydrates	31 g	Protein	10 g
	Sugar	3 g	Calcium	126 mg
	Total Fat	7.7 g	Vitamin A	436 I.U.
	Saturated Fat	1.9 g	Vitamin C	2 mg
	Cholesterol	6 mg	Folate	37 mcg
	Sodium	228 mg		

Eggplant Parmesan

Serves: 6

1 extra-large eggplant
½ cup egg substitute
⅔ cup low-salt bread crumbs
2 cups Healthy Choice® Light Roasted
    Garlic Primavera Tomato Sauce or
    similar
1 cup low-fat mozzarella cheese
Nonstick cooking spray

Peel and remove ends of eggplant. Slice into 12 slices about ¼ inch thick. Place egg substitute in small bowl and bread crumbs in a second small bowl. Coat large frying pan with nonstick cooking spray. Dip slices into egg substitute, then into breadcrumbs. Place in skillet. When slices are all placed (you probably will only be able to cook 6 at a time), begin to heat. Cook on both sides until golden brown. Coat pan again with cooking spray. Follow same instructions for remaining slices. In 2-quart (13-by-9-inch) rectangular pan coated with cooking spray, place about ½ cup of the sauce at the bottom. Layer with 6 of the eggplant slices, then ½ cup sauce, then the other 6 eggplant slices. Top with remaining sauce (1 cup) and sprinkle with cheese. Cover and bake at 350 degrees for 1 hour or until eggplant is tender and cheese is golden brown.

NUTRITIONAL ANALYSIS PER SERVING				
	Calories	134	Fiber	1 g
	Carbohydrates	17 g	Protein	10 g
	Sugar	5 g	Calcium	181 mg
	Total Fat	3.7 g	Vitamin A	814 I.U.
	Saturated Fat	1.7 g	Vitamin C	6 mg
	Cholesterol	7.8 mg	Folate	39 mcg
	Sodium	407 mg		

Indian Roasted Pork Loin with Zesty Marinade

Serves: 12

2½ pounds boneless pork loin roast
1 cup orange juice
½ cup lime juice
1¼ teaspoons ground cumin
1½ teaspoons hot pepper sauce
¾ teaspoon allspice
1 green pepper, cut into strips
1 medium onion, quartered
4 cloves garlic, finely chopped
2 packets Sweet'n Low®
NoSalt® and pepper to taste
3 teaspoons brown sugar

Remove excess fat from pork. Tenderize by pricking all over with meat fork. Place pork in plastic zip-top bag. Combine remaining ingredients except NoSalt®, pepper, and brown sugar and place in blender. Blend on medium speed until smooth. Pour mixture over pork in bag. Refrigerate, turning bag occasionally, for 4 to 20 hours. Preheat oven to 325 degrees. Remove pork from marinade and sprinkle with NoSalt® and pepper to taste. Place in shallow roasting pan. Roast uncovered for 1 to 1½ hours for medium-well. Remove from oven and let stand on platter for 15 minutes. Pour marinade into saucepan. Stir in brown sugar. Heat until it comes to a boil. Reduce heat. Stir until mixture thickens. Serve with pork.

NUTRITIONAL ANALYSIS PER SERVING				
	Calories	165	Fiber	1 g
	Carbohydrates	7 g	Protein	19 g
	Sugar	4 g	Calcium	25 mg
	Total Fat	6.5 g	Vitamin A	92 I.U.
	Saturated Fat	2.3 g	Vitamin C	23 mg
	Cholesterol	53 mg	Folate	9 mcg
	Sodium	40 mg		

Whole-Grain Veggie Lasagna

 Serves: 6

2½ cups Ragú® Light no-sugar-added
    tomato-basil sauce or similar
8 whole-wheat oven-ready lasagna
    strips
1 cup broccoli
1 cup cauliflower
1 cup part-skim ricotta cheese
½ cup low-fat mozzarella cheese
3 tablespoons grated parmesan cheese
Nonstick cooking spray

Coat a 2-quart (13-by-9) rectangular baking pan with nonstick cooking spray. Place 1 cup of sauce at bottom of pan. Layer four lasagna strips over sauce. Chop broccoli, cauliflower, and mix in ricotta and ¼ cup mozzarella cheese. Layer mixture on top of lasagna strips, cover with four more pieces of lasagna, and top with the remaining tomato sauce. Sprinkle with remaining mozzarella and parmesan cheese. Cover with foil and bake at 350 degrees for approximately 1 hour, until lasagna and veggies are soft and cheese is golden brown.

NUTRITIONAL ANALYSIS PER SERVING				
Calories	249	Fiber	7 g
Carbohydrates	31 g	Protein	15 g
Sugar	5 g	Calcium	239 mg
Total Fat	7 g	Vitamin A	618 I.U.
Saturated Fat	3 g	Vitamin C	22 mg
Cholesterol	19 mg	Folate	23 mcg
Sodium	388 mg		

Family Favorite Meat Loaf

Great for the kids.

Serves: 8

4 slices light wheat bread
1 large yellow onion, diced
2 eggs, lightly beaten
1⅓ cups frozen mixed vegetables
1 teaspoon dry mustard
1 tablespoon Worcestershire sauce
1 teaspoon NoSalt® (salt substitute)
1½ cups reduced-fat (2%) milk
2 heaping tablespoons imitation
   brown sugar
2 packets Sweet'n Low®
1 teaspoon molasses
1 tablespoon cranberry sauce
1 pound extra-lean ground beef (91%)
1 tablespoon chili sauce
Butter-flavored cooking spray

Mix all ingredients except ground beef and chili sauce. Add the ground beef by hand. Spray casserole or loaf pan with butter-flavored cooking spray. Mold meat mixture into pan. Bake at 350 degrees for 35 minutes. Spread 1 tablespoon chili sauce on top of meat loaf. Bake 10 minutes more.

NUTRITIONAL ANALYSIS PER SERVING				
	Calories	197	Fiber	2 g
	Carbohydrates	15 g	Protein	17 g
	Sugar	5 g	Calcium	91 mg
	Total Fat	7.7 g	Vitamin A	1,507 I.U.
	Saturated Fat	2.9 g	Vitamin C	3 mg
	Cholesterol	77 mg	Folate	30 mcg
	Sodium	220 mg		

Nantucket Diet Fake Fries

The kids love them!

Serves: 4

4 medium thin-skinned potatoes
Nonstick olive-oil-flavored
   cooking spray
NoSalt® (salt substitute) and pepper
   to taste
8 tablespoons low-salt ketchup
   (2 tablespoons per serving)

Place potatoes in saucepan. Cover with water. Bring to a boil and cook until just tender. (Do not overcook.) Drain and let potatoes cool. Remove skin and slice into the shape of french fries. Coat a cookie sheet with cooking spray. Arrange potato strips on cookie sheet. Bake at 375 degrees until golden brown on both sides. Season to taste and serve with low-salt ketchup.

NUTRITIONAL ANALYSIS PER SERVING					
	Calories	198	Fiber	5 g
	Carbohydrates	45 g	Protein	5 g
	Sugar	9 g	Calcium	31 mg
	Total Fat	0.7 g	Vitamin A	317 I.U.
	Saturated Fat	0 g	Vitamin C	46 mg
	Cholesterol	0 mg	Folate	39 mcg
	Sodium	19 mg		

Nantucket Diet Baked Beans

B *Serves:* 8

1 cup dry navy beans
5 cups water
¾ cup chopped onion
3 tablespoons molasses
½ cup sugar-free maple syrup
1 tablespoon Dijon mustard

Rinse beans. Place them in a saucepan with 3 cups of water. Bring to a boil. Reduce heat and simmer 2–3 minutes. Remove from heat, cover, and let soak for 1 hour. Rinse and drain beans. Place beans in an oven-safe casserole dish. Add onion, molasses, maple syrup, mustard, and 1 cup water. Mix well. Bake covered at 325 degrees for 2 hours, mixing periodically. Add remaining cup of water and cook 2 more hours or until beans are tender and the sauce is rich and thick.

NUTRITIONAL ANALYSIS PER SERVING				
Calories	125	Fiber	7 g
Carbohydrates	26 g	Protein	6 g
Sugar	5 g	Calcium	59 mg
Total Fat	0.4 g	Vitamin A	0 I.U.
Saturated Fat	0.1 g	Vitamin C	2 mg
Cholesterol	0 mg	Folate	99 mcg
Sodium	76 mg		

Cauliflower Italienne

Serves: 2

2 cups cauliflower
½ cup light spaghetti sauce (Healthy
   Choice®, Ragú®, or similar)
2 tablespoons grated parmesan or
   romano cheese

Lightly boil or steam cauliflower—do not overcook. Drain and place in oven-safe dish. Cover with sauce and cheese. Bake for 10 minutes at 375 degrees, until cheese is golden brown.

NUTRITIONAL ANALYSIS PER SERVING				
Calories	72	Fiber	4 g
Carbohydrates	11 g	Protein	5 g
Sugar	6 g	Calcium	97 mg
Total Fat	1.5 g	Vitamin A	235 I.U.
Saturated Fat	0.9 g	Vitamin C	49 mg
Cholesterol	4 mg	Folate	58 mcg
Sodium	291 mg		

Green Beans Almandine

Serves: 4

1 pound green beans
⅓ cup squeezable nonfat margarine
½ cup slivered almonds
Salt Sense® (salt substitute, 33% less
   sodium per teaspoon), and white
   pepper to taste

Wash the beans well; snip off ends. Cut into 1½-inch pieces. Boil about 10–12 minutes in small amount of salted water in covered pan. Beans should be tender. Drain well.

Heat margarine in saucepan and add the almonds. Cook until margarine is light brown. Do not burn. Toss the beans with the almond mixture and season with Salt Sense® and white pepper.

NUTRITIONAL ANALYSIS PER SERVING				
	Calories	140	Fiber	5 g
	Carbohydrates	12 g	Protein	5 g
	Sugar	2 g	Calcium	79 mg
	Total Fat	8.7 g	Vitamin A	689 I.U.
	Saturated Fat	0.6 g	Vitamin C	16 mg
	Cholesterol	0 mg	Folate	44 mcg
	Sodium	21 mg		

DESSERT

Light Cannoli

B

Serves: 8

2 ounces semisweet baking chocolate
8 premade cannoli shells
7½ ounces reduced-fat ricotta
7½ ounces fat-free ricotta
½ cup Splenda®
2 tablespoons confectioner's sugar
1 teaspoon vanilla extract
¾ cup imitation fat-free or light
   whipped topping

Place chocolate in mug. Microwave for 1–2 minutes or until chocolate melts. Dip ends of cannoli shells in chocolate and place on wax paper to cool. Let ricotta stand in strainer in refrigerator until liquid has drained out, about 1½ hours. Blend cheese with all other ingredients. Fill shells with cheese mixture. Refrigerate until set.

NUTRITIONAL ANALYSIS PER SERVING	Calories	167	Fiber	0 g
	Carbohydrates	18 g	Protein	6 g
	Sugar	5 g	Calcium	90 mg
	Total Fat	7.4 g	Vitamin A	46 I.U.
	Saturated Fat	3.2 g	Vitamin C	0 mg
	Cholesterol	16 mg	Folate	1 mcg
	Sodium	70 mg		

Fantastic Fudge Cake

*When frosted, this cake is perfect for a birthday cake,
especially if you double the layers.*

Serves: 12

1 cup soy flour
⅓ cup unsweetened cocoa powder
1½ teaspoons baking powder
1 teaspoon baking soda
¾ teaspoon cinnamon
¼ teaspoon NoSalt®
1¼ cups packed brown sugar
1 egg
2 egg whites
3 tablespoons canola oil
1 teaspoon vanilla
½ teaspoon almond extract
1 cup lowfat sour cream
Nonstick butter-flavored cooking
    spray
Fudge Frosting (optional)

Preheat oven to 350 degrees.

In a small bowl, combine flour, cocoa, baking powder, baking soda, cinnamon, and NoSalt®. Set aside.

In a medium bowl, blend brown sugar, egg, egg whites, and oil with an electric mixer on medium speed. Add the vanilla, almond extract, and sour cream. Beat on low speed until blended. Gradually add flour mixture to sour cream mixture, beating on medium speed.

Spray an 8-by-8-inch pan with nonstick butter-flavored cooking spray. Spread batter into pan. Bake for about 40 minutes or until toothpick comes out clean. Remove from oven. Cool in pan for 45 minutes. Frost with Fudge Frosting if desired.

NUTRITIONAL ANALYSIS PER SERVING	Calories	192	Fiber	2 g
	Carbohydrates	27 g	Protein	5 g
	Sugar	23 g	Calcium	91 mg
	Total Fat	8.1 g	Vitamin A	104 I.U.
	Saturated Fat	2.3 g	Vitamin C	0 mg
	Cholesterol	25 mg	Folate	30 mcg
	Sodium	189 mg		

Fudge Frosting

A

¾ cup powdered sugar

2 tablespoons unsweetened cocoa

1½ tablespoons margarine (Benecol® or similar)

1 ounce low-fat cream cheese

1¼ teaspoons fat-free half-and-half

¾ teaspoon vanilla

Beat all ingredients well and spread on cooled cake.

NUTRITIONAL ANALYSIS PER SERVING	Calories	48	Fiber	0 g
	Carbohydrates	8 g	Protein	0 g
	Sugar	7 g	Calcium	5 mg
	Total Fat	1.7 g	Vitamin A	80 I.U.
	Saturated Fat	0.5 g	Vitamin C	0 mg
	Cholesterol	1 mg	Folate	1 mcg
	Sodium	21 mg		

Jo's Biscotti

*From the Copley Seven Model Agency—a cookie that
even models will eat!*

Serves: 20 (1 cookie per serving)

1 cup all-purpose flour
1 cup confectioner's sugar
1 teaspoon baking powder
½ cup lightly toasted blanched
    almonds
½ teaspoon lemon zest
½ teaspoon cinnamon
Dash nutmeg
½ teaspoon almond extract
1 medium egg plus ½ egg white,
    slightly beaten

Preheat oven to 350 degrees. Line baking sheet with parchment paper
and set aside. Combine all dry ingredients in a large bowl, making a
small well in the middle. Add extract to egg and add to well of dry ingredients and mix by hand. Form into a log approximately 10 by 3 inches.
Lightly flatten log to about 2 inches. Place log on parchment-lined baking sheet. Bake for about 20 minutes or until top of log is slightly brown
and firm to touch. Remove from oven and let cool on a rack for 30–35
minutes. Turn oven down to 200 degrees or warm. Transfer cooled log
to a cutting board, cut ½-inch slices crosswise with a serrated knife.

Arrange slices, cut side down, on baking sheet without parchment. Bake for about 40 minutes. Remove from oven and cool completely. The biscotti can be stored in an airtight container for approximately 2 weeks. *Variation:* Add any of the following: ¼ cup pistachio nuts and ¼ coarsely chopped figs, or ¼ cup semisweet or dark chocolate coarsely chopped with ¼ cup chopped dates; substitute vanilla extract for almond and use orange zest instead of lemon, or leave out (additions will change the nutritional analysis).

NUTRITIONAL ANALYSIS PER SERVING	Calories	71	Fiber	1 g
	Carbohydrates	12 g	Protein	2 g
	Sugar	6 g	Calcium	25 mg
	Total Fat	2 g	Vitamin A	11 I.U.
	Saturated Fat	0.2 g	Vitamin C	0 mg
	Cholesterol	9 mg	Folate	14 mcg
	Sodium	29 mg		

Creamy Strawberry Cheesecake

Serves: 8

½ cup graham cracker crumbs
2 tablespoons Benecol® Light
    margarine
1 cup low-fat cottage cheese
1 8-ounce container light cream cheese
1 8-ounce container fat-free cream
    cheese
¾ cup Splenda®
2 tablespoons all-purpose flour
2 teaspoons vanilla extract
3 eggs
¼ cup skim milk
Nonstick cooking spray
Topping: 1 tablespoon confectioner's
    sugar

1½ tablespoons Splenda® (sugar
   substitute)
1 cup fresh strawberries, sliced

Spray 8-inch springform pan well with nonstick cooking spray. Melt
margarine. Stir together graham cracker crumbs and melted margarine.
Press into the bottom of the pan. Set aside. Place cottage cheese in large
bowl. Beat until smooth. Add light and nonfat cream cheese, ¾ cup
Splenda®, flour, and vanilla extract and mix until smooth. Add eggs and
mix again. Add skim milk and stir until all ingredients are combined.
Place mixture into pan. Bake at 375 degrees for 40 minutes. Cool for 30
minutes, then remove the sides of the pan. Cover and chill. For topping,
mix 1 tablespoon confectioner's sugar and Splenda® in small bowl.
When cheesecake is completely chilled, arrange sliced strawberries on
top. Sprinkle sugar mixture over the entire cheesecake.
Variation: Substitute fresh blueberries, raspberries, peaches, or bananas
for strawberries.

NUTRITIONAL ANALYSIS PER SERVING				
	Calories	213	Fiber	1 g
	Carbohydrates	15 g	Protein	14 g
	Sugar	6 g	Calcium	127 mg
	Total Fat	9.8 g	Vitamin A	866 I.U.
	Saturated Fat	4.5 g	Vitamin C	12 mg
	Cholesterol	96 mg	Folate	34 mcg
	Sodium	491 mg		

Almond Sponge Cake

Serves: 8

2 eggs
2 egg whites
⅓ cup Splenda®
1 tablespoon sugar
2 tablespoons canola oil

1 tablespoon vanilla extract
¾ cup all-purpose flour
¼ tablespoon baking soda
½ teaspoon white vinegar
Nonstick cooking spray
Frosting for Sponge Cake (optional)

Preheat oven to 350 degrees. Spray and flour a 9-inch cake pan. In a saucepan, place ½ cup water. Heat over medium heat until water is simmering.

Place mixing bowl on top of saucepan, not touching water. Add the eggs, egg whites, Splenda®, and sugar. Whisk until eggs are foamy and slightly warm. Add the oil and use an electric mixer to mix eggs until they are very foamy. Remove from heat. Add vanilla. Transfer ingredients to a larger bowl and beat the eggs until tripled in volume (about 7 minutes on high speed). Combine flour and baking soda. With a wooden spoon or spatula, fold flour and baking soda combination into whipped eggs slowly and gently. Pour the vinegar into the batter and fold in. Pour batter into pan. Bake 20–25 minutes until toothpick comes out clean. Cool before removing from pan. Frost if desired.

NUTRITIONAL ANALYSIS PER SERVING	Calories	96	Fiber	0 g
	Carbohydrates	12 g	Protein	4 g
	Sugar	2 g	Calcium	9 mg
	Total Fat	3.1 g	Vitamin A	61 I.U.
	Saturated Fat	0.5 g	Vitamin C	0 mg
	Cholesterol	53 mg	Folate	28 mcg
	Sodium	71 mg		

Frosting for Sponge Cake

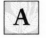

A

¾ cup confectioner's sugar
½ cup Splenda®

2 tablespoons melted Benecol®
   or similar
1 teaspoon almond or vanilla extract

Beat all ingredients and spread on cake.

NUTRITIONAL ANALYSIS PER SERVING	Calories	70	Fiber	0 g
	Carbohydrates	13 g	Protein	0 g
	Sugar	11 g	Calcium	0 mg
	Total Fat	2.3 g	Vitamin A	125 I.U.
	Saturated Fat	0.3 g	Vitamin C	0 mg
	Cholesterol	0 mg	Folate	0 mcg
	Sodium	28 mg		

Pineapple Upside-Down Cake

Serves: 8

1 can (14 ounces) crushed pineapple in
   juice, drained
2 tablespoons lemon juice
¼ cup Splenda®
1 teaspoon cornstarch
4 tablespoons soft margarine
½ cup Splenda®
1 egg
1 cup cake flour
1½ teaspoons baking powder
½ teaspoon baking soda
¼ teaspoon ground cinnamon
¼ teaspoon ground nutmeg
½ teaspoon ground ginger
⅓ cup low-fat buttermilk
Nonstick butter-flavored cooking
   spray

Preheat oven to 350 degrees. Spray baking pan with nonstick cooking spray. Drain pineapple, reserving ¼ cup juice. Mix pineapple and 1 tablespoon lemon juice, ¼ cup Splenda®, and cornstarch in bottom of 8-inch square or 9-inch round pan. Spread evenly in pan. Beat margarine and ½ cup Splenda® in medium bowl until fluffy. Beat in the egg. Combine flour, baking powder, baking soda, and spices in small bowl, then add to margarine mixture alternately with buttermilk, reserved pineapple juice, and 1 tablespoon lemon juice; begin and end with dry ingredients. Spread batter over pineapple mixture in cake pan. Bake for about 25 minutes or until toothpick tests clean when inserted in cake. Invert immediately onto serving plate and serve.

NUTRITIONAL ANALYSIS PER SERVING	Calories	150	Fiber	1 g
	Carbohydrates	23 g	Protein	3 g
	Sugar	9 g	Calcium	77 mg
	Total Fat	5.4 g	Vitamin A	304 I.U.
	Saturated Fat	0.8 g	Vitamin C	7 mg
	Cholesterol	27 mg	Folate	19 mcg
	Sodium	246 mg		

Light Tiramisu

C   *Serves:* 12

1 cup all-purpose flour
1 teaspoon baking powder
2 eggs
1 cup plus 3 tablespoons Splenda®
½ cup low-fat (1%) milk
3 tablespoons margarine (Benecol® or similar)
½ cup water
2 tablespoons light brown sugar
1 tablespoon instant coffee crystals
1 tablespoon vanilla extract

8 ounces light cream cheese
½ cup powdered sugar, sifted
1 12-ounce container fat-free or light
   whipped topping
1 tablespoon unsweetened cocoa powder
Fat-free, sugar-free chocolate sauce

Stir together flour and baking powder and set aside. Beat eggs in a bowl with electric mixer on high speed for 5 minutes. Gradually add 1 cup Splenda®, beating on medium speed for 5 minutes until fluffy. Add flour mixture and beat on low just until combined. Heat milk and margarine in a small saucepan until margarine is melted. Add to batter, beating until combined. Pour batter into a greased and floured 1½-to-2-quart glass baking dish. Bake at 350 degrees for 20 to 25 minutes until toothpick inserted comes out clean. Cool in pan on wire rack for 10 minutes.

Combine the water, 3 tablespoons Splenda®, light brown sugar, and instant coffee crystals in a small saucepan. Cook over medium heat until mixture boils. Boil for 1 minute. Remove from heat; stir in vanilla extract and set aside. Beat the cream cheese and powdered sugar. Fold in half of the whipped topping; set the remaining topping aside.

Slice cake into 12 slices, leaving the cake in the baking dish. Drizzle the coffee mixture all over the cake. Spread with the cheese mixture. Sift ¾ tablespoon cocoa powder over the cheese mixture. Drizzle the rest of the coffee mixture over the cocoa powder. Spread the remaining whipped topping over all. Drizzle with fat-free, sugar free chocolate sauce and sift the remaining ¼ tablespoon cocoa powder over finished product. Refrigerate for 4 hours before serving.

NUTRITIONAL ANALYSIS PER SERVING				
	Calories	210	Fiber	0 g
	Carbohydrates	30 g	Protein	4 g
	Sugar	13 g	Calcium	67 mg
	Total Fat	6.3 g	Vitamin A	422 I.U.
	Saturated Fat	2.7 g	Vitamin C	0 mg
	Cholesterol	45 mg	Folate	24 mcg
	Sodium	191 mg		

Healthy Chocolate Chip Cookies

B *Serves:* 18 (1 cookie per serving)

8 tablespoons Benecol® or similar
   margarine
¼ cup dark brown sugar
1 cup Splenda®
2 eggs
1 teaspoon vanilla
½ cup whole-wheat flour
½ cup all-purpose flour
½ teaspoon NoSalt® (salt substitute)
½ teaspoon baking soda
2 scoops protein powder
½ cup semisweet chocolate chips
Nonstick cooking spray

Mix all ingredients except chocolate chips and cooking spray. Fold in the chips. Coat 2 baking sheets with nonstick cooking spray. Spoon the dough onto sheets, about 1½ tablespoons per cookie, placed 2 inches apart. Bake at 350 degrees for 12–15 minutes, until golden.

Tip: You want to find a protein powder that is low in calories, carbohydrates, fat, and sugar and is high in protein. Nature's Plus® Keto Slim has only 100 calories in 2 scoops, 2 carbohydrates, 0 fat, and 0 grams of sugar. It also contains 23 grams of protein.

NUTRITIONAL ANALYSIS PER SERVING				
Calories	119	Fiber	1 g
Carbohydrates	13 g	Protein	3 g
Sugar	7 g	Calcium	8 mg
Total Fat	6.4 g	Vitamin A	250 I.U.
Saturated Fat	1.7 g	Vitamin C	0 mg
Cholesterol	24 mg	Folate	10 mcg
Sodium	93 mg		

Dining Out

JARED'S AT THE JARED COFFIN HOUSE

Jared Coffin, one of the wealthiest shipowners of his time, built the island's first three-story mansion on Broad Street in 1845. The structure has had a long history, and it is now an elegant full-service inn run by vice president and general manager John Cowden. Jared's is located within this historic building. Executive chef Cody Hixon and pastry chef Paul Terranova are masters at presenting creative local cuisine.

Seared Nantucket Bay Scallops with Cranberry Papaya Salsa

 Serves: 4

1 pound scallops
1 ripe papaya, peeled, seeded, and
    diced
½ medium red onion, chopped
½ cup sun-dried cranberries
¼ cup coarsely chopped cilantro
2 tablespoons fresh lime juice
1 clove garlic, minced or pressed
⅛ teaspoon pepper
2 teaspoons vegetable oil

Rinse the scallops and pat dry; set aside. In a medium bowl, combine papaya, red onion, cranberries, cilantro, lime juice, garlic, and pepper. Mix gently to avoid mashing the papaya. Cover and chill (will keep up to 2 days). Sear the scallops in a very hot nonstick pan with the oil. Do not move or shake the pan until the scallops start to caramelize. Spread the fruit salsa in the middle of the plate. Place scallops on top of salsa.

NUTRITIONAL ANALYSIS PER SERVING	Calories	196	Fiber	2 g
	Carbohydrates	22 g	Protein	20 g
	Sugar	12 g	Calcium	55 mg
	Total Fat	3.3 g	Vitamin A	960 I.U.
	Saturated Fat	0.3 g	Vitamin C	55 mg
	Cholesterol	37 mg	Folate	54 mcg
	Sodium	186 mg		

Pan-Seared Crab Cakes

*This recipe is actually a blend of southern deviled crab and the traditional Mary-
land crab cake. It is highly spiced with sherry, curry, paprika, and pepper, and it
is bound with very little bread to let you enjoy the crabmeat itself. Calories are
low due to replacing egg yolks with the whites and cutting back on the mayonnaise.*

Serves: 6

1¼ ounces white bread (35 g, approximately 1½ slices)
3 egg whites
1 tablespoon mayonnaise
1½ tablespoons fresh lemon juice
1½ teaspoons Worcestershire sauce
1 teaspoon dry sherry
3 drops Tabasco (or any other hot
   sauce)
1¼ teaspoons paprika
¼ teaspoon curry powder
⅛ teaspoon black pepper
½ teaspoon dry mustard
¼ teaspoon allspice
¼ teaspoon cayenne
3 teaspoons chopped fresh parsley

1¾ pounds jumbo lump crab meat
(pick over well to remove shell
pieces)
3 teaspoons olive oil

Grind bread in food processor to make bread crumbs and set aside. In medium bowl, mix egg whites, mayonnaise, lemon juice, Worcestershire, sherry, Tabasco, paprika, curry, black pepper, mustard, allspice, cayenne, and parsley. Add bread crumbs and mix well. Gently add crabmeat, handling gently so as to not break up the lumps of meat. Form into patties and chill for 30 minutes. In a nonstick pan over medium heat, add olive oil and sear the patties for about 2½ to 3 minutes on each side.

NUTRITIONAL ANALYSIS PER SERVING	Calories	186	Fiber	0 g
	Carbohydrates	6 g	Protein	26 g
	Sugar	1 g	Calcium	68 mg
	Total Fat	5.7 g	Vitamin A	437 I.U.
	Saturated Fat	0.8 g	Vitamin C	8 mg
	Cholesterol	78 mg	Folate	72 mcg
	Sodium	448 mg		

Pineapple-Raspberry Napoleon

Serves: 4

1 fresh pineapple
½ cup Yogurt Cheese (recipe follows)
1 pint fresh raspberries or blueberries
1 tablespoon confectioner's sugar

Remove top and bottom of pineapple. Place upright and slice off sides (skin) to make a square. Slice the pineapple lengthwise into 6 even pieces, cutting away the core as you slice. Stack the slices and cut them in half.

Spread 2 teaspoons yogurt cheese on top of one of the slices of pineapple and top with raspberries to cover. Repeat twice to make 3 layers per serving, ending with raspberries. Sprinkle with confectioner's sugar.

Yogurt Cheese

1 cup low-fat plain yogurt

Set a colander over a bowl and line it with a layer of paper towels. Pour the yogurt into the colander and chill, covered, for 2 hours, or until thick.

NUTRITIONAL ANALYSIS PER SERVING				
	Calories	139	Fiber	6 g
	Carbohydrates	30 g	Protein	5 g
	Sugar	20 g	Calcium	139 mg
	Total Fat	1.2 g	Vitamin A	113 I.U.
	Saturated Fat	0.4 g	Vitamin C	59 mg
	Cholesterol	4 mg	Folate	31 mcg
	Sodium	53 mg		

BRANT POINT GRILL AT THE WHITE ELEPHANT HOTEL

Brant Point Grill is highly acclaimed as Nantucket's premier lobster, steak, and seafood restaurant, and has been honored with the Wine Spectator's *Award of Excellence for the past four years. The spectacular harborside setting at the landmark White Elephant Hotel offers the ideal backdrop for the unique "Fire Cone" grill, a twenty-first-century interpretation of a Native American cooking technique. The grill tantalizes diners with dramatic visual displays while imparting a smoked mesquite flavor and unsurpassed tenderness to entrées. The Brant Point Grill skillfully concocts classic New England favorites using the freshest ingredients, enhancing them through simple preparations to maximize flavor.*

Grilled Dry-Aged New York Strip Steak with Cranberry Steak Sauce

A "Make Love to Life" Meal

Serves: 4

4 4-ounce dry-aged New York strip
  steaks
¼ cup olive oil
Salt and pepper
1 large Spanish onion, diced small
¼ cup garlic, finely chopped
1 small can peeled tomatoes
1 cup dried cranberries
2 cups cranberry juice
¼ cup coffee
¼ teaspoon cayenne
1 teaspoon hot chili powder
1 ounce (2 tablespoons) Worcestershire sauce
½ ounce (1 tablespoon) sherry vinegar

Sweat onions and garlic until soft. Add tomatoes and dried cranberries and simmer for 45 minutes or until most of the liquid is reduced. Add cranberry juice and simmer for 30 minutes. Add the rest of the ingredients and puree in a blender. You may serve this at any temperature that you prefer; I like room temperature the best. This recipe will make a little more than you need but will also keep in the refrigerator for 5 weeks.

Light the grill and let the flames die down. Never put anything on the grill until you just have glowing embers. Season the steaks with salt and pepper, then lightly brush them with the olive oil. They should not be dripping wet with oil, as this will produce charring flames from the coals. Cook the steaks to the desired doneness and place on individual plates. Serve with steak sauce over the steaks or on the side. Enjoy this with your favorite vegetable. I enjoy corn on the cob (grilled or boiled) or grilled asparagus and mashed potatoes.

NUTRITIONAL ANALYSIS PER SERVING	Calories	541	Fiber	2 g
	Carbohydrates	55 g	Protein	23 g
	Sugar	42 g	Calcium	85 mg
	Total Fat	27 g	Vitamin A	328 I.U.
	Saturated Fat	7.0 g	Vitamin C	66 mg
	Cholesterol	69 mg	Folate	12 mcg
	Sodium	297 mg		

Mixed Berries with Balsamic Vinegar and Crème Fraiche

Serves: 4

3 cups mixed berries, preferably
    strawberries cut into quarters and
    raspberries
½ to 1 ounce (1 to 2 tablespoons)
    25–50-year-old balsamic vinegar
    (the older the vintage, the less you
    will need)
1 tablespoon turbinado sugar
Pepper to taste
⅓ cup crème fraiche, found in grocery
    or specialty stores

Combine the first three ingredients in a bowl, gently toss, and let sit for
10 minutes. Add pepper to taste and toss again. Divide into 4 individual
bowls and then top with crème fraiche.

NUTRITIONAL ANALYSIS PER SERVING	Calories	127	Fiber	4 g
	Carbohydrates	14 g	Protein	1 g
	Sugar	9 g	Calcium	41 mg
	Total Fat	7.9 g	Vitamin A	315 I.U.
	Saturated Fat	4.6 g	Vitamin C	49 mg
	Cholesterol	27 mg	Folate	26 mcg
	Sodium	13 mg		

THE CHANTICLEER

Jean-Charles Berruet, owner and chef extraordinaire of the world-famous Chanticleer in the tiny village of Siasconset on Nantucket, creates an incomparable culinary experience for his diners.

Established in 1970, the Chanticleer has become one of the world's most renowned restaurants. The cuisine is traditional French with an emphasis on local fruits and vegetables as well as products from the sea. The Chanticleer's magnificent wine cellar boasts more than 40,000 bottles of fine wine. The Wine Spectator *has given the restaurant its Grand Award every year since 1987, and* Lifestyles of the Rich and Famous *lists it as one of the top ten most romantic restaurants in the world.*

Beignets de Bluefish Timgad

Serves: 5

2 pounds bluefish, filleted and cut into
   thick scallopini
1 cup water
5 tablespoons olive oil
4 cloves garlic
2 hot peppers
1 lemon, peel only
1 tablespoon coriander seed
1 tablespoon cumin
1 pinch saffron
2 tablespoons grated ginger
6 mint leaves
1 pound tomatoes, peeled, seeded, and
   chopped
1 cup fish stock
¼ cup flour
2 eggs
Salt and pepper to taste

In blender, make marinade with 1 cup water, 3 tablespoons olive oil, garlic, hot peppers, lemon peel, coriander seed, cumin, saffron, ginger, and mint leaves. Marinate the bluefish scallopini for a few hours.

Sauté the chopped tomato in 1 tablespoon of olive oil. Add fish stock, 1 cup of the marinade, and salt to taste. Cook for 15 minutes. Blend until smooth; set aside and keep warm. Take scallopini out of marinade and add salt and pepper to taste. Dredge in flour and then dip in beaten egg. Sauté the scallopini in 1 tablespoon olive oil for 2 minutes on each side. Serve with the tomato sauce.

NUTRITIONAL ANALYSIS PER SERVING	Calories	389	Fiber	3 g
	Carbohydrates	13 g	Protein	33 g
	Sugar	4 g	Calcium	62 mg
	Total Fat	22.6 g	Vitamin A	1,589 I.U.
	Saturated Fat	3.9 g	Vitamin C	42 mg
	Cholesterol	165 mg	Folate	44 mcg
	Sodium	193 mg		

Poulet aux Abricots (*Braised Chicken with Dried Apricots*)

A "Make Love to Life" Meal

Serves: 10

2 pounds chicken, cut in pieces
21 ounces dried apricots, soaked in
   water for one hour
2 tablespoons olive oil
3 onions, sliced
2 cloves garlic, chopped
½ teaspoon allspice
1 lemon, sliced
½ teaspoon ginger powder

Salt and pepper to taste
1 teaspoon chopped fresh coriander
Cooked brown rice for serving

Sauté the onions in oil for about 5 minutes. Add the garlic, allspice, and ginger. Sauté the chicken pieces in oil, browning them on all sides. Put the chicken on top of the onions and add the lemon slices. Season with salt and pepper. Add ½ cup water. Cover and cook for 30 minutes. Add apricots and cook for another 30 minutes. Add the coriander and cook for another 10 minutes. (Optional) Serve with cooked brown rice, ½ cup (not included in analysis), adds 110 calories.

NUTRITIONAL ANALYSIS PER SERVING				
	Calories	348	Fiber	5 g
	Carbohydrates	43 g	Protein	14 g
	Sugar	28 g	Calcium	57 mg
	Total Fat	13.3 g	Vitamin A	557 I.U.
	Saturated Fat	3.3 g	Vitamin C	22 mg
	Cholesterol	48 mg	Folate	5 mcg
	Sodium	48 mg		

TOPPER'S AT THE WAUWINET INN

Rated as one of North America's finest restaurants, Topper's at the 1876 Wauwinet Inn, a member of the prestigious association of Relais & Châteaux, offers an extraordinary world-class dining experience with a Nantucket sensibility.

Topper's award-winning wine list is a repeated recipient of the coveted Wine Spectator's *Grand Award and the* Wine Enthusiast's *Award of Excellence, providing the perfect accompaniment to chef Chris Freeman's signature cooking style, which celebrates Nantucket's native seafood and local delicacies.*

Bluefin Tuna Carpaccio with Soba Noodle and Pickled Vegetable Salad

 D

Serves: 6

18 ounces #1 grade bluefin tuna
½ package (4.4 ounces) soba noodles,
   cooked, cooled, and tossed with
   ¼ cup sesame oil
½ cup shredded carrots
½ cup julienned red pepper
½ cup julienned yellow pepper
½ cup green onion, stalks only,
   cut thin on the bias
3 cloves garlic, minced
½ tablespoon patis (Asian fish sauce)
½ teaspoon Tabasco sauce
½ cup rice wine vinegar
1 tablespoon sugar
2 tablespoons flying fish roe
Salt and pepper to taste
24 sprigs cilantro
2 tablespoons julienned pickled ginger
1 tablespoon cracked coriander
2 bunches upland cress or watercress
2 tablespoons chopped chives

Cut tuna into ¼-inch-thick pieces. Place between 2 pieces of plastic wrap. Gently flatten tuna to ¹⁄₁₆ inch with meat pounder. Keep covered until ready to assemble.

Combine carrots, peppers, green onion, garlic, patis, Tabasco, rice wine vinegar, and sugar and bring to a boil. Chill and hold until ready to serve. Arrange three pieces of tuna on each plate. Combine soba noodles, vegetable mixture, chives, and upland cress. Season with salt and pepper. Place noodle salad on top of tuna in center. Top with pickled ginger. Arrange cilantro around salad and sprinkle with cracked coriander and flying fish roe.

NUTRITIONAL ANALYSIS PER SERVING	Calories	323	Fiber	2 g
	Carbohydrates	21 g	Protein	26 g
	Sugar	4 g	Calcium	98 mg
	Total Fat	15.1 g	Vitamin A	4,846 I.U.
	Saturated Fat	2.6 g	Vitamin C	48 mg
	Cholesterol	63.7 mg	Folate	19 mcg
	Sodium	392 mg		

Steamed Littleneck Clams with Champagne, Roma Tomatoes, and Scallions

 Serves: 6

2 tablespoons extra-virgin olive oil
1 tablespoon minced garlic
6 Roma tomatoes, peeled, seeded, and
    diced
2 cups Champagne
72 littleneck clams, washed (no bro-
    ken shells)
1 bunch scallions, washed and sliced
    on bias
2 tablespoons chopped Italian parsley
Fresh cracked black pepper to taste

Heat a large pan. Add olive oil and minced garlic. Sauté to release aroma. Add tomatoes and sauté 1 minute. Add Champagne and bring to a simmer. Add littleneck clams and scallions. Cover pot with a lid. As clams open, remove them from the pot and place into a large bowl. When all clams are open and removed, add chopped parsley and season with black pepper. Pour liquid over clams and serve.

NUTRITIONAL ANALYSIS PER SERVING	Calories	207	Fiber	2 g
	Carbohydrates	11 g	Protein	16 g
	Sugar	4 g	Calcium	87 mg
	Total Fat	5.9 g	Vitamin A	1,820 I.U.
	Saturated Fat	0.8 g	Vitamin C	38 mg
	Cholesterol	37 mg	Folate	51 mcg
	Sodium	75 mg		

AMERICAN SEASONS

Perennially at the top of the "not-to-be-missed" list, American Seasons special-izes in contemporary regional American cuisine and has been described by Zagat's as the most creative food on the island. Executive chef Michael LaScola and wife Orla's personal twist on cuisine and their groundbreaking dishes con-tinually delight their patrons.

Pesto-Crusted Rack of Lamb

D

Serves: 10

1 full large rack of lamb (our preference is Australian)
3 tablespoons olive oil
1½ cups pesto (recipe follows)
3 carrots
2 onions
½ stalk celery
Salt and pepper to taste

Preheat the oven to 375 degrees. Trim the excess fat from the lamb and clean the bones. Put the olive oil in a sauté pan and heat on high. Season the lamb with salt and pepper. Place the lamb meat side down in pan and sear till golden. Remove from the pan and set the rack to one side. Clean and roughly chop the carrots, onions, and celery. Place them in a roast-ing pan and place the meat bone side down on top of vegetables. Thickly coat the meat with pesto (recipe to follow) and place in oven. Roast for

15 minutes or longer, depending on how well done you prefer your meat. Remove from oven and rest meat for 10 minutes. Slice into chops and serve.

NUTRITIONAL ANALYSIS PER SERVING (WITHOUT PESTO)				
Calories	367	Fiber	3 g
Carbohydrates	10 g	Protein	28 g
Sugar	3 g	Calcium	127 mg
Total Fat	24.3 g	Vitamin A	4,227 I.U.
Saturated Fat	7.2 g	Vitamin C	11 mg
Cholesterol	84 mg	Folate	21 mcg
Sodium	176 mg		

Pesto

B

Serves: 10

½ pound basil
½ pound baby spinach
6 large cloves garlic
¼ cup extra-virgin olive oil
¼ cup pine nuts
½ cup parmesan
1 teaspoon sugar
Salt and pepper to taste

Place all the ingredients in a food processor and blend until fairly smooth.

NUTRITIONAL ANALYSIS PER SERVING				
Calories	108	Fiber	2 g
Carbohydrates	5 g	Protein	3 g
Sugar	1 g	Calcium	99 mg
Total Fat	9 g	Vitamin A	2,016 I.U.
Saturated Fat	2 g	Vitamin C	8 mg
Cholesterol	4 mg	Folate	17 mcg
Sodium	99 mg		

Mélange of Truffled Petite Spring Vegetables

Serves: 12

1 bunch baby leeks
2 bunches baby carrots
1 bunch candy-striped beets (or regu-
    lar beets)
1 bunch golden beets
1 pound shelled English spring peas
1 cup peeled red pearl onions
2 bunches baby white turnips
2 bunches asparagus
1 clove minced garlic
1 teaspoon black truffle oil
3 tablespoons butter
1 bunch fresh basil, finely chopped
1 cup chicken stock
Salt and pepper to taste
2 tablespoons canned black truffle
    slices

Clean and trim all the vegetables. Blanch in salted boiling water, then cool quickly in iced water. Using a large sauté pan over medium heat, melt the butter and add the truffle oil. Sauté the garlic lightly. Remove the vegetables from the cold water and dry them. Add to the sauté pan, ensuring that all vegetables are lightly coated with the pan mixture. Add the chicken stock and basil. Season with salt and pepper. Allow all the vegetables to warm through. Put the vegetables in a warmed serving dish and garnish with truffle slices. Serve immediately.

NUTRITIONAL ANALYSIS PER SERVING	Calories	151	Fiber	7 g
	Carbohydrates	25 g	Protein	6 g
	Sugar	13 g	Calcium	74 mg
	Total Fat	4 g	Vitamin A	3,370 I.U.
	Saturated Fat	1.6 g	Vitamin C	21 mg
	Cholesterol	8 mg	Folate	225 mcg
	Sodium	159 mg		

THE LASCOLAS' PHILOSOPHY AND DINING TIPS

Orla and Michael LaScola believe that the body needs some of all types of food, fresh and organic when possible. They stress that people should eat what they need in moderation. They feel that everyone should pay more attention to the source of their food: "If individuals can gain knowledge of food, it will hopefully bring about a healthier way of eating." The LaScolas advocate the following dining-out tips:

- *Look at the food on tables around you. Determine portion sizes and order accordingly.*
- *Know your sauces: demiglace, for example, will have less fat than butter-based sauces. If you eat a butter sauce, just do not finish it, and take a walk in the morning.*
- *Just because you pay for it does not mean that you need to finish it!*

CAMBRIDGE STREET RESTAURANT

Brandt Gould is the founding chef and owner of Cambridge Street Restaurant on Nantucket Island. Gould built Cambridge Street in 1994 as a modest bar and grill to "ensure that I had a place that I would like to go to." It has since grown and morphed into a lively full-service restaurant with three dining rooms, an outdoor patio, and a constantly evolving menu of fresh foods from around the world.

Originally from the Midwest and trained as an artist (painter/sculptor) in Massachusetts, Brandt first came to Nantucket to cook during college as a way to pay for school. It was during those days that he first developed the recipe for his trademark Nantucket Longneck BBQ Sauce.

Babaghanouj

 Serves: 6

2 medium eggplant
1 tablespoon tahini (more or less to
   taste)
¼ cup olive oil or vegetable oil
3 peeled garlic cloves
2 tablespoons lemon juice
½ teaspoon salt
1 or 2 sprigs parsley, chopped
   (optional)

Halve the two eggplant lengthwise. Place them cut side down on a lightly oiled sheet pan. Roast at 400–425 degrees for approximately 40 minutes; rotate at 20-minute intervals. The flesh of the eggplant should be soft, caramel-colored, and easy to scoop out with a fork or spoon, not crispy or burned. In a large bowl mix together the tahini and olive oil, then very finely puree together the garlic and scooped-out eggplant flesh. Mix in the lemon juice, salt, and parsley. It should be smooth and easy to pick up with a toasted piece of pita bread. It should taste rich with a slight tang, with enough salt to call you back for more. Play with all the ingredients until you find that perfect balance for yourself.

NUTRITIONAL ANALYSIS PER SERVING				
Calories	134	Fiber	0 g
Carbohydrates	10 g	Protein	2 g
Sugar	0 g	Calcium	20 mg
Total Fat	10.6 g	Vitamin A	44 I.U.
Saturated Fat	1.5 g	Vitamin C	6 mg
Cholesterol	0 mg	Folate	37 mcg
Sodium	201 mg		

Cambridge Street's Grilled Yellowfin Tuna with Chunky Pineapple Salsa and Spicy Asian Slaw

When making this dish, it is very important to start with fresh tuna from your fish market, preferably not from a supermarket. What you are looking for is fish that is rich pink to burgundy red and firm and resilient to the touch. It should smell pleasantly of the sea, not overly fishy. If you cannot get a piece of fresh fish, a frozen piece is great—in fact, sometimes better. Ask the clerk at the fish market for a 1-pound chunk of tuna. This can be sliced lengthwise into four blocks that will be about 1 inch thick and 5 inches long. Make sure that the skin and the deep purple blood lines are removed before using. Tuna is a good source of omega-3 fatty acids. Grilling or dry-searing fish is so much better than deep-frying.

Serves: 16

TUNA RUB

> 1½ cups sesame seeds, white or mixed
> 1 cup flaked nori (chop by hand or use
>   a coffee grinder)
> ¾ cup flaked dulse
> 2½ teaspoons anise or fennel seed,
>   crushed
> 2 tablespoons black pepper
> 1 teaspoon dried coriander
> 1 tablespoon sesame oil

Mix all ingredients except oil and set aside.

PINEAPPLE SALSA

> 1 pineapple, peeled and sliced
> 2 Anaheim or cubanelle peppers
> 1 chili pepper

½ Spanish onion, sliced
1 tablespoon prepared chipotle,
   chopped
1 tablespoon vegetable or olive oil
2 tablespoons molasses
2 tablespoons soy sauce
2 tablespoons rice wine vinegar
1 cucumber, seeded and diced
Salt and pepper to taste

Grill first four ingredients until charred, then chop thoroughly. Toss with remaining ingredients and set aside.

ASIAN SLAW

1 head Napa cabbage
1 bunch bok choy
¼ cup black or white sesame seeds
2 teaspoons pickled hot peppers (deli
   style), minced
¾–1 cup rice wine vinegar
¼ cup sesame oil

Cut light feathery pieces off the top of the cabbage and bok choy using a dramatic 45-degree angle. The pieces should be about bite-sized and delicate like fallen leaves. In a large bowl, add sesame seeds, peppers, vinegar, and sesame oil; toss.

PULLING IT ALL TOGETHER

This is best if the tuna is cooked on the grill, but you can do it in a hot dry skillet or carefully beneath a broiler. First, dip the blocks of tuna in a shallow dish of sesame oil, just to coat them. Then drop each piece into the rub mix to coat, and set aside on a clean plate. When all are coated, drop onto a hot grill and cook on each surface for about a minute and a half, maybe less, maybe more, depending on your equipment. This is when you realize that it would be nice to have a little extra piece of tuna to perform a test with. The finished tuna should be cooked only enough for the rub to be seared in place and the center of the block to be warmed. If it is cooked too long, it will crack and flake apart when cut.

With a sharp knife cut each block of fish into ½-inch-thick cross sections and fan them out decoratively on each plate like you might see in a sushi restaurant. The fish should at this point look like an order of sushi, with the concentric patterns visible. Arrange the salsa and the slaw on either side and serve with tamari sauce and wasabi paste to taste. Cold or warm sake is an excellent companion for this dish, but any favorite wine or full-bodied beer will do nicely.

NUTRITIONAL ANALYSIS PER SERVING	Calories	493	Fiber	9 g
	Carbohydrates	31 g	Protein	32 g
	Sugar	13 g	Calcium	272 mg
	Total Fat	29.7 g	Vitamin A	6,369 I.U.
	Saturated Fat	4.1 g	Vitamin C	123 mg
	Cholesterol	38 mg	Folate	143 mcg
	Sodium	489 mg		

BRANDT GOULD'S PHILOSOPHY AND DINING TIPS

As far as health and nutrition are concerned, Brandt upholds a philosophy of balance and moderation while also subscribing to Chinese physiological principles that employ certain components of diet for specific health gains. However, food is but a fragment of a life that is to be enjoyed; the more that one consumes of good clean legumes and grains with less meats and fried or processed foods, then the more one can develop a taste for all the elements in life that are truly beneficial to the body and the spirit.

SFOGLIA

Sfoglia's philosophy of the dining experience is a time-honored tradition of cooking the freshest, most local food available in a simple, straightforward manner and bringing it to the table to share with family and friends. Italians have an enormous respect for food and take their mealtimes very seriously. While meals may span several courses, they are always consumed in moderation.

Chefs and owners Ron and Colleen Suhanosky have created a menu that is designed for healthy eating in moderation. Always using seasonal ingredients, most appetizers are fruit- and vegetable-based, and portion sizes are realistic.

Pasta dishes can be ordered in half or full-size portions, and entrees are served without sides, which can be ordered separately. This allows the diner the option to tailor a meal according to his or her own specifications.

Sfoglia Mussels

Serves: 2–4

1 tablespoon olive oil
1 tablespoon julienned salami
1 pound mussels, cleaned
1 teaspoon ground fennel
1 teaspoon hot pepper (or less)
¼ cup white wine
½ cup chopped parsley
4 plum tomatoes (canned San
    Marzano or best quality), crushed

In a large braising pot heat oil and toast salami lightly. Add mussels and toss to coat. Add fennel, hot pepper, white wine, parsley, and crushed plum tomatoes. Cover tightly and let steam 5–8 minutes or until opened. Serve in warm bowls with all the juices poured over the top.

NUTRITIONAL ANALYSIS PER SERVING				
	Calories	143	Fiber	2 g
	Carbohydrates	8 g	Protein	4 g
	Sugar	4 g	Calcium	46 mg
	Total Fat	9.1 g	Vitamin A	2,067 I.U.
	Saturated Fat	1.5 g	Vitamin C	55 mg
	Cholesterol	7 mg	Folate	48 mcg
	Sodium	192 mg		

Watermelon and Tomato Salad

B   *Serves:* 4

2 Large Brandywine or Beefsteak
   tomatoes, room temperature, sliced
8 thin slices watermelon
Salt and pepper to taste (sea salt is
   best)
4 tablespoons mixture of basil, tarragon, parsley
4 tablespoons extra-virgin olive oil
Juice of 1 or 2 lemons

Arrange sliced tomato and watermelon on 4 plates, alternating between fruit and tomato. Season with salt and pepper. Snip herbs over tomato and watermelon (about 1 tablespoon per plate). Drizzle with extra-virgin olive oil (about 1 tablespoon per plate) and a squeeze of lemon juice to taste. Serve immediately.

NUTRITIONAL ANALYSIS PER SERVING				
Calories	168	Fiber	2 g
Carbohydrates	13 g	Protein	2 g
Sugar	9 g	Calcium	27 mg
Total Fat	13.9 g	Vitamin A	1,654 I.U.
Saturated Fat	1.9 g	Vitamin C	30 mg
Cholesterol	0 mg	Folate	27 mcg
Sodium	11 mg		

Whole-Wheat Spaghetti with Lemon, Almond, and Dandelion Greens

 Serves: 10

1 pound whole-wheat spaghetti
3 tablespoons plus ¼ cup olive oil
½ onion, chopped
½ bunch dandelion greens, chopped
    roughly
.15 ounces (a pinch) of pepperoncini
    (hot pepper), chopped
½ cup white wine
Salt and pepper to taste
Zest of 1 lemon
¾ cup chopped almonds, toasted
¼ cup chopped parsley
4 tablespoons grated parmigiano reg-
    giano
10 tablespoons ricotta

Slowly cook onion in 3 tablespoons olive oil until soft and translucent. Add greens, season with salt, pepper, and pepperoncini, cover, and steam until tender. Add wine; reduce by half. Meanwhile, boil spaghetti until al dente. Pour into large bowl; add greens, lemon zest, almonds, and parsley. Toss with remaining ¼ cup olive oil and dust with parmigiano reggiano. Serve in warm bowls with a dollop of ricotta, 1 tablespoon per bowl.

NUTRITIONAL ANALYSIS PER SERVING				
Calories	348	Fiber	7.2 g
Carbohydrates	37.6 g	Protein	11.2 g
Sugar	2.4 g	Calcium	129.6 mg
Total Fat	17.6 g	Vitamin A	1,010 I.U.
Saturated Fat	3.2 g	Vitamin C	9.6 mg
Cholesterol	8 mg	Folate	20 mcg
Sodium	65.6 mg		

THE SUHANOSKYS' PHILOSOPHY AND DINING TIPS

Dining out can be a challenge, especially for those trying to main-tain healthy eating habits. We recommend ordering the simplest dishes, steering clear of food that is too contrived or that too many hands have touched. Generally, these dishes are far removed from their natural state. Ordering one entrée between two people allows you to taste but not feel obligated to clean the plate. Soups are always great fillers, especially broth-based ones, and always nourishing. Limit bread intake—bread should be eaten with your meal as an accompaniment, not as an appetizer alone. Fruit or sorbets are great ways to finish a meal, leaving you satisfied, not stuffed.

SEAGRILLE

The Seagrille is a very popular spot for year-round island residents, as well as the summer crowd. The restaurant offers an extensive menu of exquisite seafood dishes, including their renowned clam chowder, and a variety of selec-tions from the land. Chef/owner E. J. Harvey's culinary expertise offers dishes that will tempt every palate, including the kids'.

Roasted Pesto-Crusted Striped Bass with Farm Tomato and Tat Soi Salad

A *"Make Love to Life"* Meal

Serves: 4

1 cup Japanese bread crumbs (panko)
6 ounces prepared pesto
2 ounces melted butter
4 6-ounce filets striped bass
1 large red farm tomato

1 bunch asparagus
Dash salt
Dash pepper
1 tablespoon olive oil
1 large red farm tomato
8 ounces tat soi (Asian greens; any
    mixed greens can be used)
8 ounces low-calorie vinaigrette dress-
    ing

Combine the bread crumbs, pesto, and butter. Coat the bass filets individually. Roast in oven at 400 degrees for 13 minutes or to desired doneness. While the bass is cooking, trim asparagus and season with salt,
pepper, and olive oil. Grill asparagus on outdoor barbecue. Slice the
tomatoes and arrange on plate, alternating the different colors of tomatoes. Toss tat soi with vinaigrette and place on top of tomato. Place finished bass on top. Lean the asparagus on the bass. Drizzle with a little
vinaigrette.

NUTRITIONAL ANALYSIS PER SERVING				
	Calories	684	Fiber	4 g
	Carbohydrates	30 g	Protein	42 g
	Sugar	5 g	Calcium	420 mg
	Total Fat	44.1 g	Vitamin A	3,310 I.U.
	Saturated Fat	13 g	Vitamin C	26 mg
	Cholesterol	182 mg	Folate	158 mcg
	Sodium	1,652 mg		

THE TUCKERNUCK INN CAFÉ

*The Tuckernuck Inn Café provides the ideal mix of quality and value. Owned
by Jack and Laddy McElderry, this bistro-style eatery at the Tuckernuck Inn has
a small dining room that offers a tranquil summer escape. Its ambiance is casual
and welcoming, and the cuisine is delectable. The entrées aren't overly fancy and
are cooked in ways that showcase their fresh ingredients. The wine list of more
than 120 wines mirrors this harmony of simplicity and excellence.*

Tuckernuck Inn Café
Paper Bag Catch

Serves: 4

4 6-ounce salmon filets or thick white
    fish filets
8 tablespoons lemon juice
2 teaspoons finely chopped ginger
    (optional)
Salt and pepper to taste
2 tablespoons extra-virgin olive oil
3 red potatoes, boiled until just tender
    and sliced thin
1 cup snow peas, blanched and
    drained
2 carrots, thinly sliced, blanched and
    drained
1 small zucchini, thinly sliced
Handful of cherry tomatoes
Chopped dill, basil, or thyme
Nonstick cooking spray

Preheat oven to 400 degrees. Cut a standard-size brown paper bag so
you have just the bottom half. Spray bag with cooking spray. Put all
ingredients in bag and roll bag down so it is closed. Cook for 20–25
minutes or until fish is tender. Cut around the top of the bag to retain the
juices. Serve with mixed greens.

Variation: Any vegetables may be substituted as long as you blanch
harder vegetables first. The recipe can also be done in foil packets if bags
are not available; cooking time may vary by 5 minutes or so.

NUTRITIONAL ANALYSIS PER SERVING	Calories	376	Fiber	3 g
	Carbohydrates	17 g	Protein	36 g
	Sugar	5 g	Calcium	57 mg
	Total Fat	17.9 g	Vitamin A	4,306 I.U.
	Saturated Fat	2.6 g	Vitamin C	54 mg
	Cholesterol	94 mg	Folate	89 mcg
	Sodium	107 mg		

Tuckernuck Inn Café Cappuccino Cheesecake

A "Make Love to Life" Dessert

Serves: 12

1½ cups ground chocolate cookie
    crumbs (I use icebox cookies)
6 tablespoons butter
1½ cups semi-sweet chocolate pieces
32 ounces cream cheese, softened
⅔ cup sugar
¼ cup whole milk
3 eggs
⅓ cup espresso powder
½ teaspoon cinnamon
Nonstick cooking spray

Heat the oven to 350 degrees.

Combine cookie crumbs and melted butter and press into a 9-inch springform pan sprayed with cooking spray. Press cookie crumbs only about 1 inch up the side. Melt the chocolate in a double boiler over low heat, stirring constantly. In mixer, combine cream cheese and sugar in large bowl on medium speed until blended. Use the paddle attachment on the mixer if you have one. Add milk, eggs, espresso powder, and cinnamon and beat until well blended. Add melted chocolate and mix until blended. Make sure there is no cream cheese mixture stuck on the bottom. Spoon mixture into crust and gently tap pan to remove any air bubbles. Place foil around pan just in case the pan leaks. Bake 55 minutes or until top is not soft. Remove and place on cooling rack for 15 minutes. Run a knife around the side of the pan and remove side first. Cool for at least 4 hours before serving. Slice and serve with whipped cream and shaved chocolate.

NUTRITIONAL ANALYSIS PER SERVING				
Calories	540	Fiber	2 g
Carbohydrates	37 g	Protein	9 g
Sugar	27 g	Calcium	83 mg
Total Fat	41.6 g	Vitamin A	1,255 I.U.
Saturated Fat	24.2 g	Vitamin C	0 mg
Cholesterol	151 mg	Folate	25 mcg
Sodium	366 mg		

COMPANY OF THE CAULDRON

If you want to feel as if you have your own private chef, make reservations to dine at Company of the Cauldron. Located in the heart of Nantucket's historic district, the charming, romantic setting and outstanding creative cuisine make for a perfect dining choice.

Proprietors All and Andrea Kovalencik design elegant menus offered each evening as a prix fixe dinner.

The name was given to the restaurant as a tribute to the first cooking academy established in Florence since Roman times, called Company of the Cauldron.

Polenta-Crusted Swordfish with Avocado Chutney

Serves: 10

3½ pounds swordfish, cut 2 inches
    thick
¼ cup olive oil
1 cup instant polenta, ground fine
1 teaspoon cumin, seed
1 teaspoon ground coriander, seed
½ teaspoon garlic powder
Salt and pepper to taste
2 tomatoes, seeded and chopped
2 whole avocados, pitted and diced
1 small red onion, chopped fine
Juice of 1½ key limes
3 ears corn, kernels removed from cob
½ cup black beans cooked in stock,
    until just tender
1 tablespoon rice wine vinegar
1 tablespoon brown sugar
1 bunch scallions, chopped
1 bunch cilantro, chopped fine

Cut swordfish into ten 2-inch pieces. Combine half of the spices with all
of the polenta in a mixing bowl including salt and pepper. Rub swordfish with a little olive oil (1 tablespoon) and dredge in polenta mixture.
Mix the tomatoes, chopped avocados, red onion, lime juice, and the rest
of the spices and set the chutney aside. Pan-sear the swordfish polenta
side down over high heat in 2 tablespoons olive oil for 3 to 4 minutes.
Bake at 400 degrees until just cooked through. Reheat the black beans
and corn together in 1 tablespoon olive oil with the rice wine vinegar,
brown sugar, and chopped scallions, and season to taste. Make a traditional hollandaise but with key lime juice instead of lemon (recipe to follow). Warm dinner plate; spread the black beans in the center. Place

swordfish on beans; top fish with some of the chutney and a dab of hollandaise. Garnish with a fresh sprig of cilantro. Serve immediately.

Hollandaise Sauce

¾ cup water plus 2 tablespoons
A pinch of salt, paprika, red pepper,
    and dry mustard
2 tablespoons fresh key lime juice
1 tablespoon cornstarch
2 egg yolks
3 tablespoons butter

Place water in a double boiler. Heat water, salt, paprika, red pepper, dry mustard, and lime juice. Dissolve cornstarch in 2 tablespoons of water. Add to seasoned water and stir constantly. Remove from heat when mixture begins to thicken. Beat egg yolks and stir them into mixture. Add 1 tablespoon of butter. Mix and place over hot water until thickened. Add remaining butter and serve.

NUTRITIONAL ANALYSIS PER SERVING WITHOUT HOLLANDAISE				
	Calories	596	Fiber	6 g
	Carbohydrates	30 g	Protein	37 g
	Sugar	5 g	Calcium	50 mg
	Total Fat	37.4 g	Vitamin A	2,012 I.U.
	Saturated Fat	15.3 g	Vitamin C	18 mg
	Cholesterol	172 mg	Folate	85 mcg
	Sodium	182 mg		

Cisco Stout Marinated Filet Mignon

A "Make Love to Life" Meal

Serves: 4

4 6-ounce filet mignons
1 quart Cisco Stout (from Nantucket's
    Cisco Brewers)
1 cup brown sugar
1 medium onion, chopped
4 tablespoons balsamic vinegar
4 tablespoons French mustard
3 tablespoons thyme, chopped
3 tablespoons Worcestershire sauce
3 cloves garlic, chopped
1 tablespoon kosher salt
1 tablespoon black pepper
¼ cup olive oil

Combine all ingredients except the stout in a blender; slowly add the beer while blending. Marinade should be sweet and tangy, with the fresh thyme coming through. Marinate the filets for three hours. Brush with olive oil, salt, and pepper. Grill on high heat for two minutes per side; give each side a half turn halfway through cooking. Finish in the oven at 450 degrees until desired doneness is reached.

NUTRITIONAL ANALYSIS PER SERVING				
Calories	578	Fiber	0 g
Carbohydrates	16 g	Protein	30 g
Sugar	15 g	Calcium	35 mg
Total Fat	42.6 g	Vitamin A	24 I.U.
Saturated Fat	16.3 g	Vitamin C	2 mg
Cholesterol	121 mg	Folate	12 mcg
Sodium	522 mg		

CIOPPINO'S

Cioppino's was founded in 1990 by the husband-and-wife team of Susan and Tracy Root. Located in an old Nantucket home situated in the heart of the downtown historic district, this elegant restaurant offers an eclectic menu with an impressive wine list. Cioppino's is known to islanders as the place to dine when looking for fine food in an atmosphere of casual refinement.

Tomato Bisque

 Serves: 12

1 14.5-ounce can whole tomatoes
1 cup olive oil
2 onions
1 small piece ginger
12 cloves garlic, roasted
2 tablespoons paprika
2 14.5-ounce cans diced tomato
1 gallon chicken stock or broth
3 cups chopped fresh basil

Drain whole tomatoes (reserve juice), lightly coat with some of the olive oil, then roast at high heat for 10 to 15 minutes in a medium stockpot. Set aside. Sauté onions with ginger in the remaining olive oil until translucent; add garlic, paprika, and diced tomatoes, and mix evenly. Add chicken stock and juice from whole tomatoes, then crush the roasted tomatoes and add to the pot. Simmer 45 minutes to 1 hour. Season to taste and add basil. Serve cold.

NUTRITIONAL ANALYSIS PER SERVING	Calories	314	Fiber	3 g
	Carbohydrates	20 g	Protein	10 g
	Sugar	10 g	Calcium	61 mg
	Total Fat	22.1 g	Vitamin A	1,425 I.U.
	Saturated Fat	3.5 g	Vitamin C	14 mg
	Cholesterol	10 mg	Folate	27 mcg
	Sodium	588 mg		

Spiced Nuts

A *"Make Love to Life"* Snack

D

Serves: 32 (¼-cup servings)

3 ounces brandy
2 tablespoons ginger puree
3 cups brown sugar
½ cup honey
2 tablespoons Cajun spice
4 pounds nuts

Preheat oven to 350 degrees. Flame brandy and combine with ginger puree, brown sugar, and honey, stirring over low heat until sugar is completely dissolved. Add remaining ingredients and remove from heat. Spread in a single layer onto sheet pan and bake for 15–20 minutes. Remove from oven and work with spatula until cool.

NUTRITIONAL ANALYSIS PER SERVING	Calories	385	Fiber	5 g
	Carbohydrates	26 g	Protein	10 g
	Sugar	11 g	Calcium	46 mg
	Total Fat	29.2 g	Vitamin A	9 I.U.
	Saturated Fat	3.9 g	Vitamin C	0 mg
	Cholesterol	0 mg	Folate	29 mcg
	Sodium	111 mg		

FOG ISLAND CAFÉ

At Fog Island Café, owners Mark and Anne Dawson, both graduates of the Culinary Institute of America, have created a casual, inviting atmosphere with an emphasis on hospitality.

Fog Island is open year-round, offering high-quality, delectable dishes in season for breakfast, lunch, and dinner. The restaurant's mission statement is to deliver a menu of healthy products with value and quality as a priority. They believe that every customer should receive a "feel-good feeling" and be served with speed and systematic precision so that they will want to return often.

Chicken Soup

Many islanders go to Fog Island in the winter just for the soup.

Serves: 8

2½ pounds boneless, skinless chicken
1 pound chopped fresh vegetables (for veggie soup, increase vegetables and eliminate chicken), for example, ½ cup carrots, ½ cup celery, ½ cup green peas, ½ cup mushrooms
1 small can diced green chili peppers, undrained
3 cups water
2 low-sodium chicken bouillon cubes
1 small can Italian-style diced tomatoes, undrained
1 teaspoon ground cumin
1 teaspoon coriander
Pepper to taste
3 cups dry pasta shells, cooked

Place all items except pasta into a large pot, stir, and bring to a boil. Reduce heat to low and simmer for 20–30 minutes. Add cooked pasta, heat through, and serve.

NUTRITIONAL ANALYSIS PER SERVING	Calories	310	Fiber	3 g
	Carbohydrates	25 g	Protein	34 g
	Sugar	6 g	Calcium	61 mg
	Total Fat	7.7 g	Vitamin A	3,065 I.U.
	Saturated Fat	1.9 g	Vitamin C	20 mg
	Cholesterol	61.5 mg	Folate	85.5 mcg
	Sodium	461 mg		

Fog Style Chicken Hash

A "Make Love to Life" Meal

This unusual breakfast dish has become an island favorite.

Serves: 8

2 tablespoons clarified butter
1 cup diced onion
½ cup diced green pepper
½ cup diced red pepper
1 tablespoon minced garlic
½ teaspoon salt
1 teaspoon paprika
½ teaspoon black pepper
½ teaspoon white pepper
½ teaspoon thyme
½ teaspoon chili powder
4 cups poached and diced chicken meat
3 cups boiled and diced red bliss potatoes

½ cup sliced scallions
½ cup chopped parsley
1 cup light half and half
12 eggs, poached
6 to 12 slices whole-grain bread,
   toasted

Melt the butter in a large sauté pan or skillet over medium heat. Add the onions, peppers, and garlic and cook until tender. Add the seasonings and cook for 1 minute to toast the spices. Stir in the poached chicken meat, potatoes, scallions, parsley, and cream. Taste the hash and adjust the seasoning to taste. Continue to cook, stirring occasionally, until the cream reduces and the hash becomes golden brown in color. Flip the hash over and brown the other side as well. Remove from the heat and portion onto warmed serving plates. Top each serving of hash with two freshly poached eggs and serve with 1 to 2 slices of toast.

NUTRITIONAL ANALYSIS PER SERVING				
	Calories	518	Fiber	5 g
	Carbohydrates	45 g	Protein	45 g
	Sugar	9 g	Calcium	146 mg
	Total Fat	20.9 g	Vitamin A	1,887 I.U.
	Saturated Fat	7.7 g	Vitamin C	50 mg
	Cholesterol	514 mg	Folate	89 mcg
	Sodium	748 mg		

THE DAWSONS' PHILOSOPHY AND DINING TIPS

Mark and Anne Dawson believe that eating right and exercising are equally important factors in staying healthy.

STRAIGHT WHARF

The Straight Wharf Restaurant, with its location directly on the waterfront, has been considered a must for serious wine and food lovers for twenty-seven years. Executive chef Steve Cavagnaro creates an amazing menu focusing on Mediterranean-inspired local seafood, simply and elegantly prepared, accom-

panied by island-grown produce and herbs from the restaurant's own herb garden.

The Straight Wharf's wine list has been honored with the Wine Spectator's *Best of Award of Excellence. Great French burgundies, rare and older vintages, and small producers attract wine lovers from among locals and visitors alike.*

The dining room is very Nantucket. The weathered shingle walls are awash with candlelight and hung with the delightful work of island artists. The water-front deck is a magnificent setting for al fresco dining. In addition to the dining room, the harborside bar/café is a great spot for more casual dining; it's the place to be for a late-night goombay smash or apple martini.

Seared Shrimp with Vegetable Spring Rolls and Lemongrass

 Serves: 6

18 large fresh shrimp (31–35 per
  pound), peeled and deveined
2 sprigs lemon thyme
8 basil leaves
1 small onion
1 stalk celery, thinly sliced
1 garlic clove, minced
1½ inches ginger, minced
2 stalks lemongrass, thinly sliced
2 carrots, peeled and thinly sliced
2 red bell peppers, thinly sliced
2 lime leaves (optional), chopped
1 pint chicken stock
4 tablespoons grapeseed oil or other
  neutral oil
Sea salt and black pepper to taste
1 lime

Prepare Vegetable Spring Rolls (recipe follows) and set aside. Rinse shrimp. Remove heads, peel, and devein. Set aside.

To make sauce, reserve the heads and shells. Chop coarsely. Cut a 20-by-40-inch square of cheesecloth. Wrap the reserved shrimp shells, basil, and lemon thyme in the cheesecloth and tie as a sachet.

To a medium saucepot add 1 tablespoon of the grapeseed oil and over low heat begin to sweat the onion, celery, garlic, ginger, and lemongrass. Cook until onion is translucent. Add the red pepper, carrots, and lime leaves. Raise heat to medium and cook for 3 minutes to soften vegetables.

Add the chicken stock. Raise heat and bring broth to boil, then lower heat and simmer 30 minutes. Add sachet and continue simmering 15 minutes. Remove sachet. Correct seasoning with salt and pepper. Allow broth to cool slightly, then puree until smooth and pass through a chinois or similar fine strainer. Season with fresh lime juice. Set aside.

To serve, gently reheat sauce. Rewarm spring rolls in 225 degree oven to recrisp. Season shrimp with salt and pepper. Add 3 tablespoons grapeseed oil to sauté pan. Over medium-high heat, cook shrimp 1½ minutes a side. Remove shrimp, blot on absorbent paper, and finish plating.

Vegetable Spring Rolls

Makes 8 rolls

1 ounce packed bean threads
2 ounces, (4 tablespoons) toasted
   sesame oil
1 small leek, julienned
1 tablespoon minced garlic
1¼ tablespoons minced ginger
1 teaspoon minced chili pepper
2–3 small carrots, peeled and julienned
2 stalks celery, peeled and julienned
1 large red pepper, seeded and
   julienned
1 small zucchini, julienned
2 cups sliced shiitake mushrooms

1 cup bean sprouts
2 cups Napa cabbage, thinly sliced
½ ripe mango, peeled and julienned
2 scallions, green part only, sliced
Salt and pepper to taste
8 small rice papers
1 cup canola oil or peanut oil

Rehydrate bean threads by cooking quickly in boiling water. Strain and shock in ice water. Strain and reserve.

Heat 1 teaspoon of sesame oil in wok or sauté pan until fragrant. Add leeks, garlic, ginger, and chili pepper; sauté until leeks are crisp and tender. Spread mixture on sheet pan or plate to cool.

Cook the remaining vegetables, individually, in a similar manner and cool each one with the others.

Once all the vegetables have been cooked and cooled, combine them in a large bowl with the bean threads, mango, and scallions. Season with salt and pepper. Gently squeeze out extra liquid from vegetable filling.

To assemble the spring rolls, soak the rice papers in a large bowl of hot tap water just until the edges soften. Remove the rice papers, shake off the excess water, and lay them flat on a work surface. When the rice paper becomes pliant, blot up any excess water and spoon ⅛ of filling onto the paper. Fold each side toward the center and roll away from the bottom to enclose the mixture. Pull gently on the rice paper to ensure a tight roll. To cook, heat canola or peanut oil in a small pan to 350 degrees. Fry until golden brown, gently turning the spring rolls. Remove and drain on absorbent paper.

NUTRITIONAL ANALYSIS PER SERVING				
	Calories	457	Fiber	5 g
	Carbohydrates	38 g	Protein	10 g
	Sugar	11 g	Calcium	93 mg
	Total Fat	31.4 g	Vitamin A	7,232 I.U.
	Saturated Fat	2.9 g	Vitamin C	143 mg
	Cholesterol	34 mg	Folate	69 mcg
	Sodium	214 mg		

Paillards of Striped Bass Sautéed with Mesclun Greens and Virgin Tomato Sauce

 Serves: 8

Virgin Tomato Sauce

6 medium ripe tomatoes, peeled,
   seeded, chopped into ¼-inch dice
2 cloves garlic, peeled and minced
2 tablespoons lemon juice
5 tablespoons extra-virgin olive oil
2 tablespoons, fresh, cleaned and dry
   basil
Coarse salt
Freshly ground black pepper

Lightly salt the diced tomato and place in a strainer with a bowl under-neath to collect the tomato water. Reserve water for another use; allow the tomatoes to drain for 15 minutes. Mix in ceramic bowl the tomato and the remaining ingredients. The sauce is ready but is better if given one or two hours to ripen in covered bowl at room temperature. Whip sauce just before serving.

Mesclun Greens

Approximately 4 cups young dandelion
   leaves, frisee or curly endive, lime-
   stone bibb, mache, baby bok choy,
   arugula, peppercress, radicchio,
   lovage, sorrel, and/or nasturtium

leaves and flowers (according to
your taste and seasonal availability)
1 teaspoon thyme
2 tablespoons lemon thyme
1 teaspoon minced rosemary
1 teaspoon minced pineapple sage
1 tablespoon minced tarragon
2 teaspoons minced chives
2 tablespoons chervil
2 tablespoons minced basil
1 tablespoon minced mint
1 tablespoon minced Italian parsley
2 tablespoons sherry vinegar
6 tablespoons extra-virgin olive oil
Kosher salt to taste
Fresh black pepper to taste

Wash and dry the greens very carefully. Tear the leaves by hand into a
bowl. Refrigerate until serving time, to crisp and refresh the salad.

Into the salad bowl, add all of the herbs. Toss the salad with salt,
pepper to taste, and add the sherry vinegar, continuing to toss thoroughly but gently. Add the olive oil. Taste for seasoning.

Striped Bass

8 pieces of fresh striped bass, approximately ½ inch thick and weighing
2–3 ounces each
3 teaspoons coarsely ground coriander
seed
2 teaspoons coarsely ground green
peppercorns
½ teaspoon kosher salt
1 tablespoon canola oil

Season the striped bass on one side with coriander seeds, green peppercorns, and salt. Meanwhile, heat a black iron skillet or other heavy-bottomed pan over high heat for approximately 3–4 minutes. The pan should just comfortably accommodate the striped bass pieces without overlapping. Add the oil and quickly place the striped bass slices in the pan—seasoned side down. If the pan is properly hot, turn the striped bass over 15 seconds after the last piece is put in the pan. Remove all pieces after 30 seconds. Place on paper towels to remove excess oil.

Arrange the greens on a plate. Pour the sauce on the plate next to the greens. Place the striped bass across the greens.

NUTRITIONAL ANALYSIS PER SERVING				
Calories	277	Fiber	3 g
Carbohydrates	8 g	Protein	12 g
Sugar	4 g	Calcium	43 mg
Total Fat	23.5 g	Vitamin A	2,172 I.U.
Saturated Fat	3.1 g	Vitamin C	21 mg
Cholesterol	47 mg	Folate	24 mcg
Sodium	200 mg		

THE SUMMER HOUSE

The Summer House is one of the most elegant restaurants on Nantucket. Located in a beautiful part of the island called Siasconset, dining at the Summer House is a truly delightful experience. Executive chef and operator Michael Farrell specializes in contemporary American cuisine and uses only the freshest local ingredients in the Northeast. Farrell took over the restaurant in 2000. He has gained national acclaim in such publications as Zagat, DiRona, Wine Spectator, and Martha Stewart Living. His previous positions have included executive chef at both Castle Pines Country Club in Denver and Beano's Cabin in Beaver Creek, Colorado. He most recently was the executive chef who opened three dining facilities at the renowned Anthem Country Club in Las Vegas.

Curry Lemongrass Broth

B

Serves: 12

1 quart carrot juice
1 8-ounce can clam juice
2 cans Thai coconut milk
1 cup lime juice
2 stalks lemongrass
½ teaspoon curry paste
1 teaspoon curry powder
1 teaspoon whole coriander seed
2 star anise
½ cup sugar
Cornstarch

Make a paste with cornstarch and water, to be used as a thickening agent (amount varies depending upon how thick you want your broth to be) and set aside.

Combine all ingredients and simmer for 10 minutes. Thicken with cornstarch paste. Excellent for any seared seafood; goes well with Asian noodles as well.

NUTRITIONAL ANALYSIS PER SERVING				
Calories	199	Fiber	1 g
Carbohydrates	19 g	Protein	2 g
Sugar	9 g	Calcium	42 mg
Total Fat	14.3 g	Vitamin A	1,736 I.U.
Saturated Fat	12.6 g	Vitamin C	10 mg
Cholesterol	1 mg	Folate	13 mcg
Sodium	95 mg		

Cranberry Soup

A *"Make Love to Life"* Soup

 Serves: 24

6 pounds cranberries
3 quarts water
1 pound sugar
22 ounces honey
1 750-ml bottle white wine
Zest of 2 oranges
Zest of 2 limes
Zest of 2 lemons
3 cinnamon sticks
1 teaspoon whole cloves
¼ teaspoon salt
Freshly ground pepper
Lime juice

In a stainless-steel pot, combine all ingredients. Bring to a boil, then turn down heat to a low simmer and cook for 30 minutes. Turn off heat and let settle undisturbed for one hour. Strain through a large chinoise, then the fine chinoise (this is a clear soup, so do not force through).

NUTRITIONAL ANALYSIS PER SERVING				
Calories	237	Fiber	4 g
Carbohydrates	55 g	Protein	0 g
Sugar	51 g	Calcium	8 mg
Total Fat	0 g	Vitamin A	3 I.U.
Saturated Fat	0 g	Vitamin C	13 mg
Cholesterol	0 mg	Folate	1 mcg
Sodium	27 mg		

THE DOWNYFLAKE

For breakfast or lunch, the Downyflake has been satisfying the appetites of locals and visitors for over fifty years. The Downyflake is most famous for its homemade doughnuts, but regulars swear by the blueberry pancakes with homemade blueberry syrup and the cinnamon-bun French toast. Fluffy three-egg omelets are also a specialty, with many choices of meat and/or vegetable and cheese fillings.

Owners since 1999, Mark Hogan and Susan Tate have striven to uphold the humble traditions of the restaurant—good food at a fair price. The Downyflake proudly serves the year-round community, providing a place for families, working people, and visitors to enjoy breakfast and lunch in a friendly, relaxed atmosphere.

Fluffy Veggie Omelet for One

B

Serves: 1

8 ounces egg substitute
2 tablespoons chopped broccoli,
    steamed
2 tablespoons chopped mushrooms,
    steamed
2 tablespoons diced fresh tomato
2 tablespoons chopped onion, steamed
Nonstick cooking spray
1 tablespoon shredded or chopped
    parmesan

Prepare vegetables and set aside.

Beat egg substitute 30 seconds on high with a hand mixer to make omelet fluffy. Spray 8-inch nonstick skillet with cooking spray. Heat over medium-high heat until pan is hot. Add the egg substitute and cook until set but soft (2–3 minutes). Put pan under a broiler for 30 to 45 seconds until eggs are firm and completely set; this makes eggs puff up.

Remove from broiler and add cheese; return to broiler until cheese is melted (30 seconds or so). When cheese is melted, remove from broiler. Warm vegetables in microwave and put on top of omelet. Slide omelet onto a plate, folding omelet over once to cover veggies.

NUTRITIONAL ANALYSIS PER SERVING	Calories	165	Fiber	1 g
	Carbohydrates	9 g	Protein	27 g
	Sugar	6 g	Calcium	149 mg
	Total Fat	1.7 g	Vitamin A	1,676 I.U.
	Saturated Fat	0.9 g	Vitamin C	13 mg
	Cholesterol	4 mg	Folate	146 mcg
	Sodium	581 mg		

Cinnamon-Bun French Toast

A *"Make Love to Life" Breakfast*

 D

Serves: 2

2 large premade cinnamon buns (3½–4 inches in diameter)
3 eggs
½ teaspoon vanilla
1 large pinch cinnamon

If cinnamon buns are heavily frosted, scrape or cut off the sugar topping. Slice horizontally into 2 or 3 rounds, each ½ to ¾ inch thick, depending on thickness of bun. Beat egg, vanilla, and cinnamon and dip each piece in the mixture. Heat a griddle or heavy pan. When hot, grill cinnamon bun slices until nicely browned (3–4 minutes per side). Use butter or cooking spray to coat pan if not using a nonstick griddle. Top with real maple syrup.

NUTRITIONAL ANALYSIS PER SERVING (WITHOUT SYRUP)	Calories	334	Fiber	1 g
	Carbohydrates	32 g	Protein	13 g
	Sugar	19 g	Calcium	101 mg
	Total Fat	17.5 g	Vitamin A	665 I.U.
	Saturated Fat	8.3 g	Vitamin C	0 mg
	Cholesterol	37.2 mg	Folate	35 mcg
	Sodium	295 mg		

ANNYE'S WHOLE FOODS

Annye Camara has developed her natural food store to include a wide variety of selections for the health-conscious. Annye's Whole Foods has everything from grains and nuts to fresh organic produce, frozen organic foods, dairy items, healthy sweets, and vitamins and supplements. From the juice bar you can order a fabulous smoothie or protein drink made with everything from fresh seasonal fruits to nuts, dates, peanut or almond butter, yogurt, low-calorie protein powder, and even echinacea, ginseng, or flaxseed oil. You can even name your favorite smoothie and keep it on file.

Annye's Island Famous Organic Smoothie

C

¼ cup organic blueberries, frozen
¼ cup organic strawberries, frozen
½ cup bananas, frozen, or ½ cup
    organic pears
1–2 scoops protein powder (soy, rice,
    or whey)
1½ cups organic milk (soy, rice, dairy,
    or almond)

Blend all ingredients together until rich and creamy.

Tip: We suggest ingredient combinations that will provide 15–20 grams of protein, so that the smoothie makes a satisfying meal.

NUTRITIONAL ANALYSIS PER SERVING				
	Calories	288	Fiber	3 g
	Carbohydrates	24 g	Protein	24 g
	Sugar	15 g	Calcium	8 mg
	Total Fat	0.2 g	Vitamin A	36 I.U.
	Saturated Fat	0 g	Vitamin C	23 mg
	Cholesterol	0 mg	Folate	9 mcg
	Sodium	1 mg		

Simple Pleasures

This section contains recipes that can be made from start to finish in approximately 30 minutes or less.

BREAKFAST

French Toast

 Serves: 1

2 slices light bread
¼ cup egg substitute
1 packet NutraSweet®
⅛ teaspoon cinnamon
Nonstick cooking spray
2 tablespoons sugar-free maple syrup

Mix egg substitute, sweetener, and cinnamon in a bowl. Dip bread slices into mixture and place on frying pan coated with nonstick cooking spray. Cook until golden on each side. Serve with sugar-free maple syrup.

NUTRITIONAL ANALYSIS PER SERVING				
	Calories	146	Fiber	3 g
	Carbohydrates	22 g	Protein	10 g
	Sugar	2 g	Calcium	63 mg
	Total Fat	3.4 g	Vitamin A	227 I.U.
	Saturated Fat	0.8 g	Vitamin C	0 mg
	Cholesterol	1 mg	Folate	9 mcg
	Sodium	312 mg		

Nantucket Diet Fried Cinnamon Apples

Great for pancakes.

Serves: 2

2 apples, peeled and sliced
2 tablespoons squeezable nonfat mar-
    garine
¼ cup sugar-free maple syrup
1 teaspoon vanilla extract
⅛ teaspoon cinnamon

Place all ingredients in a small frying pan and cook until apples are tender and golden brown.

NUTRITIONAL ANALYSIS PER SERVING					
Calories	107		Fiber	5 g
Carbohydrates	28 g		Protein	0 g
Sugar	16 g		Calcium	2 mg
Total Fat	0 g		Vitamin A	100 I.U.
Saturated Fat	0 g		Vitamin C	5 mg
Cholesterol	0 mg		Folate	0 mcg
Sodium	48 mg			

Maple Walnut Cream of Wheat

Serves: 1

3 tablespoons Cream of Wheat instant
    hot cereal
½ cup water
½ cup skim milk

2 tablespoons sugar-free maple syrup
1½ tablespoons chopped walnuts

Place cream of wheat and water in microwave-safe bowl. Heat until cereal comes to a boil, about 2 minutes. Mix in remaining ingredients and serve.

NUTRITIONAL ANALYSIS PER SERVING	Calories	253	Fiber	2 g
	Carbohydrates	39 g	Protein	9 g
	Sugar	0 g	Calcium	242 mg
	Total Fat	7.9 g	Vitamin A	1,742 I.U.
	Saturated Fat	0.8 g	Vitamin C	0 mg
	Cholesterol	2 mg	Folate	136 mcg
	Sodium	106 mg		

Banana Oatmeal

Serves: 1

½ cup rolled oats
1 cup water
⅓ cup sliced banana
¼ cup skim milk
Artificial sweetener to taste

Place oats and water in microwave safe bowl. Cook for approximately two minutes, or until oatmeal starts to boil. Mix and add banana, milk, and sweetener.

Variation: Try topping with 2 tablespoons of dry roasted peanuts or 2 tablespoons of sugar-free maple syrup (additions will change the nutritional analysis).

NUTRITIONAL ANALYSIS PER SERVING	Calories	223	Fiber	6 g
	Carbohydrates	42 g	Protein	9 g
	Sugar	8 g	Calcium	79 mg
	Total Fat	2.7 g	Vitamin A	197 I.U.
	Saturated Fat	0.5 g	Vitamin C	4 mg
	Cholesterol	1 mg	Folate	19 mcg
	Sodium	29 mg		

Apple Cinnamon Oatmeal

Serves: 1

½ cup diced apples
⅛ teaspoon cinnamon
½ cup rolled oats
1 cup water
2 packets artificial sweetener
⅓ cup skim milk

Place diced apples, cinnamon, oats, and water in microwave safe bowl. Mix and place in microwave; cook for 1–2 minutes, until it comes to a boil. Add in sweetner, milk and serve.

Variations: Add 1 mini box raisins or 1 tablespoon, 2 tablespoons chopped dates, or 2 tablespoons almonds or walnuts (additions change analysis).

NUTRITIONAL ANALYSIS PER SERVING	Calories	230	Fiber	7 g
	Carbohydrates	44 g	Protein	9 g
	Sugar	11 g	Calcium	98 mg
	Total Fat	2.6 g	Vitamin A	258 I.U.
	Saturated Fat	0.5 g	Vitamin C	2 mg
	Cholesterol	2 mg	Folate	10 mcg
	Sodium	38 mg		

Vanilla Oatmeal

 Serves: 1

½ cup rolled oats
1 cup water
1–2 teaspoons imitation vanilla
   extract or flavoring
¼ cup skim milk
Artificial sweetener to taste

Place oats and water in microwave-safe bowl. Cook until cereal begins to boil. Mix in vanilla, milk and sweetener.

NUTRITIONAL ANALYSIS PER SERVING				
	Calories	181	Fiber	4 g
	Carbohydrates	31 g	Protein	8 g
	Sugar	2 g	Calcium	77 mg
	Total Fat	2.6 g	Vitamin A	165 I.U.
	Saturated Fat	0.5 g	Vitamin C	0 mg
	Cholesterol	1 mg	Folate	9 mcg
	Sodium	29 mg		

Cinnamon Toast

Serves: 1

2 slices light multigrain bread
1½ tablespoons Benecol® Light mar-
    garine (or similar)
1 tablespoon Splenda®
¼ teaspoon cinnamon

Toast bread. Spread margarine over both slices. Mix sweetener and cinnamon together. Sprinkle over toast.

NUTRITIONAL ANALYSIS PER SERVING				
	Calories	149	Fiber	3 g
	Carbohydrates	17 g	Protein	3 g
	Sugar	1 g	Calcium	32 mg
	Total Fat	8.8 g	Vitamin A	752 I.U.
	Saturated Fat	1.1 g	Vitamin C	0 mg
	Cholesterol	0 mg	Folate	0 mcg
	Sodium	318 mg		

LUNCH

Tuna Melt

Serves: 1

1 2.7-ounce can tuna packed in water
1 tablespoon light mayonnaise
1 tablespoon chopped celery
NoSalt® (salt substitute) and pepper to
    taste
1 slice fat-free sharp cheddar cheese
2 slices light whole-wheat bread

Mix tuna, mayonnaise, and celery. Season to taste. Place mixture on one slice of bread. Add slice of cheese and top with other slice of bread. Microwave for 20–30 seconds or until cheese is melted.

NUTRITIONAL ANALYSIS PER SERVING				
	Calories	253	Fiber	3 g
	Carbohydrates	17 g	Protein	30 g
	Sugar	2 g	Calcium	438 mg
	Total Fat	7 g	Vitamin A	352 I.U.
	Saturated Fat	1.5 g	Vitamin C	0 mg
	Cholesterol	31 mg	Folate	5 mcg
	Sodium	758 mg		

Apple Tofu Salad with Raspberry Lime Vinaigrette

Serves: 1

3 cups mixed greens
1 apple, diced
¼ package (99 grams) light tofu, cubed
2 tablespoons chopped dry-roasted
    walnuts
2 tablespoons Raspberry Lime Vinai-
    grette (recipe follows)

Place all ingredients in a salad bowl. Add dressing. Toss and serve.

NUTRITIONAL ANALYSIS PER SERVING				
Calories	242	Fiber	10 g
Carbohydrates	30 g	Protein	11 g
Sugar	18 g	Calcium	141 mg
Total Fat	11 g	Vitamin A	4,589 I.U.
Saturated Fat	1.1 g	Vitamin C	32 mg
Cholesterol	0 mg	Folate	205 mcg
Sodium	126 mg		

Raspberry Lime Vinaigrette

Serves: 20 (approximately 2 tablespoons per serving)

1 12-ounce package frozen raspberries
⅓ cup sugar-free raspberry jam
¼ cup olive oil
2 tablespoons lime juice

2 tablespoons vinegar
½ cup Splenda®
⅔ cup water

Allow raspberries to thaw. Place all ingredients in blender. Blend until smooth.

NUTRITIONAL ANALYSIS PER SERVING	Calories	41	Fiber	1 g
	Carbohydrates	5 g	Protein	0 g
	Sugar	2 g	Calcium	5 mg
	Total Fat	2.8 g	Vitamin A	6 I.U.
	Saturated Fat	0.4 g	Vitamin C	5 mg
	Cholesterol	0 mg	Folate	4 mcg
	Sodium	0 mg		

Mandarin Salad

B

Serves: 1

2 cups lettuce
¼ cup fat-free cottage cheese
½ cup canned mandarin oranges in
    their own juice
½ cup green grapes

Place all ingredients in a bowl and serve.

This salad does not really need dressing because you can use some of the natural juice of the oranges.

NUTRITIONAL ANALYSIS PER SERVING					
Calories	156		Fiber	3 g
Carbohydrates	32 g		Protein	9 g
Sugar	27 g		Calcium	100 mg
Total Fat	0.4 g		Vitamin A	4,857 I.U.
Saturated Fat	0.1 g		Vitamin C	55 mg
Cholesterol	3 mg		Folate	88 mcg
Sodium	233 mg			

Greek Salad

 B

Serves: 1

2 cups mixed greens
½ cup sliced tomatoes
6 black olives
2 tablespoons feta cheese
2 tablespoons fat-free Greek or Italian
    dressing

Combine all ingredients. Top with dressing and serve.

NUTRITIONAL ANALYSIS PER SERVING					
Calories	127		Fiber	4 g
Carbohydrates	12 g		Protein	6 g
Sugar	6 g		Calcium	193 mg
Total Fat	6.8 g		Vitamin A	3,958 I.U.
Saturated Fat	3.3 g		Vitamin C	30 mg
Cholesterol	18 mg		Folate	147 mcg
Sodium	838 mg			

Shrimp Salad with Tomato Vinaigrette

B

Serves: 1

2–3 cups mixed greens
3 ounces shrimp, boiled and chilled
¼ cup sliced red pepper
¼ cup sliced green pepper
¼ cup sliced cucumber
2 tablespoons chopped scallions
2 tablespoons Tomato Vinaigrette
    (recipe follows)

Place all ingredients in large salad bowl. Toss and top with vinaigrette (2 tablespoons approximately).

NUTRITIONAL ANALYSIS PER SERVING				
Calories	141	Fiber	4 g
Carbohydrates	11 g	Protein	20 g
Sugar	2 g	Calcium	124 mg
Total Fat	2 g	Vitamin A	4,597 I.U.
Saturated Fat	0.4 g	Vitamin C	124 mg
Cholesterol	129 mg	Folate	153 mcg
Sodium	220 mg		

Tomato Vinaigrette

Serves: 5 (approximately two tablespoons per serving)

½ cup V8® or tomato juice
1 tablespoon vinegar
½ tablespoon Mrs. Dash® Minced
   Onion Medley Seasoning
2 packets Sweet'n Low®

Combine all ingredients. Chill and serve.

NUTRITIONAL ANALYSIS PER SERVING	Calories	7 g	Fiber	0 g
	Carbohydrates	2 g	Protein	0 g
	Sugar	1 g	Calcium	4 mg
	Total Fat	0 g	Vitamin A	200 I.U.
	Saturated Fat	0 g	Vitamin C	6 mg
	Cholesterol	0 mg	Folate	0 mcg
	Sodium	62 mg		

Spinach Salad with Dijon Dressing

Serves: 1

2–3 cups fresh baby spinach leaves
2 slices reduced-fat or soy bacon
1 hard-boiled egg, sliced
½ cup sliced mushrooms

Seasoning to taste
2 tablespoons Dijon dressing (recipe
    follows)

Cook bacon until crisp. Cool and crumble. Place all ingredients in a
salad bowl. Top with Dijon dressing and bacon bits.

NUTRITIONAL ANALYSIS PER SERVING				
	Calories	179	Fiber	2 g
	Carbohydrates	8 g	Protein	14 g
	Sugar	1 g	Calcium	73 mg
	Total Fat	10.4 g	Vitamin A	3,436 I.U.
	Saturated Fat	3.4 g	Vitamin C	15 mg
	Cholesterol	224 mg	Folate	28 mcg
	Sodium	406 mg		

Dijon Dressing

Serves: 6 (2 tablespoons per serving)

6 ounces plain fat-free yogurt
2 tablespoons vinegar
1 tablespoon honey Dijon mustard
1 tablespoon yellow mustard
2 packets Sweet'n Low®

NUTRITIONAL ANALYSIS PER SERVING				
	Calories	25	Fiber	0 g
	Carbohydrates	4 g	Protein	1 g
	Sugar	3 g	Calcium	40 mg
	Total Fat	0.5 g	Vitamin A	128 I.U.
	Saturated Fat	0.1 g	Vitamin C	2 mg
	Cholesterol	1 mg	Folate	0 mcg
	Sodium	51 mg		

Caesar Salad

Serves: 1

2–3 cups romaine lettuce
2 tablespoons shredded or grated
   parmesan
2 tablespoons fat-free dressing
2 tablespoons croutons

Place lettuce in bowl. Mix in cheese and dressing. Top with croutons.
Variation: For Chicken Caesar Salad, cook 1 Perdue® low-fat breaded
chicken breast, following baking instructions on package. Slice and add
to salad. (For the Chicken Caesar Salad, the calories are 250.)

NUTRITIONAL ANALYSIS PER SERVING				
Calories	102	Fiber	3 g
Carbohydrates	11 g	Protein	7 g
Sugar	4 g	Calcium	171 mg
Total Fat	3.4 g	Vitamin A	6,548 I.U.
Saturated Fat	1.8 g	Vitamin C	27 mg
Cholesterol	9 mg	Folate	158 mcg
Sodium	668 mg		

Terrific Turkey Wrap

Serves: 1

1 honey wheat flour tortilla
3 slices fat-free turkey breast
1 tablespoon cranberry sauce
1 tablespoon light mayonnaise

¼ cup alfalfa sprouts
2 thin slices red onion

Place all ingredients on top of the wrap, roll, and enjoy.

NUTRITIONAL ANALYSIS PER SERVING				
	Calories	190	Fiber	3 g
	Carbohydrates	31 g	Protein	9 g
	Sugar	8 g	Calcium	21 mg
	Total Fat	5.8 g	Vitamin A	20 I.U.
	Saturated Fat	1.2 g	Vitamin C	2 mg
	Cholesterol	17 mg	Folate	15 mg
	Sodium	724 mg		

BLT Light

Serves: 1

2 slices light multigrain bread
3 slices reduced-fat bacon or soy
    bacon
3 or 4 lettuce leaves
3 or 4 tomato slices
1 tablespoon light mayonnaise

Place bacon in skillet. Cook until crisp. Let cool. Spread mayonnaise on slice of bread. Top with lettuce, tomato, and bacon and other slice of bread.

Variation: Try adding Dijon or honey mustard for extra flavor; adds approximately 10 calories.

NUTRITIONAL ANALYSIS PER SERVING	Calories	226	Fiber	4 g
	Carbohydrates	19 g	Protein	10 g
	Sugar	4 g	Calcium	50 mg
	Total Fat	13 g	Vitamin A	1,990 I.U.
	Saturated Fat	4 g	Vitamin C	9 mg
	Cholesterol	23 mg	Folate	43 mcg
	Sodium	661 mg		

Tuna Veggie Roll-Up

Serves: 1

1 honey wheat tortilla (45 g)
1 2.7-ounce can tuna packed in water
1 tablespoon light mayonnaise
3 tomato slices
3 or 4 slices red pepper
3 or 4 slices green pepper
¼ cup shredded lettuce
NoSalt® (salt substitute) and pepper to
    taste

Mix tuna and mayonnaise. Season to taste. Top tortilla with tuna mixture and all the veggies and roll up.

NUTRITIONAL ANALYSIS PER SERVING	Calories	231	Fiber	3 g
	Carbohydrates	25 g	Protein	23 g
	Sugar	2 g	Calcium	33 g
	Total Fat	6.3 g	Vitamin A	1,410 I.U.
	Saturated Fat	1.3 g	Vitamin C	60 mg
	Cholesterol	28 mg	Folate	23 mcg
	Sodium	558 mg		

Chicken Breast Sandwich

Serves: 1

2 slices light rye bread
6 slices chicken breast, Healthy
   Choice® Deli Thin Oven Roasted or
   similar
2 lettuce leaves
3 tomato slices
1 tablespoon fat-free Thousand Island
   dressing

Place chicken, lettuce, and tomato on one slice of bread. Top with dressing and other slice of bread.

NUTRITIONAL ANALYSIS PER SERVING				
	Calories	199	Fiber	4 g
	Carbohydrates	24 g	Protein	22 g
	Sugar	7 g	Calcium	45 mg
	Total Fat	3.3 g	Vitamin A	1,495 I.U.
	Saturated Fat	1.2 g	Vitamin C	9 mg
	Cholesterol	38 mg	Folate	33 mcg
	Sodium	814 mg		

Ham and Pickle Pita

Serves: 1

1 large 57 g whole-wheat pita
3 slices low-salt fat-free ham
1 slice fat-free cheddar cheese
¼ cup shredded lettuce
3 slices tomato
8 sugar-free low-salt bread-and-butter
   pickle slices
1 tablespoon fat-free honey Dijon
   dressing

Slice top of pita. Place all ingredients inside and serve.

NUTRITIONAL ANALYSIS PER SERVING				
Calories	286	Fiber	4 g
Carbohydrates	43 g	Protein	24 g
Sugar	7 g	Calcium	261 mg
Total Fat	3.2 g	Vitamin A	979 I.U.
Saturated Fat	1 g	Vitamin C	8 mg
Cholesterol	32 mg	Folate	21 mcg
Sodium	1,085 mg		

You can reduce the sodium to 570 mg by deducting the cheese and pickles. The calories will also lower to 175.

DINNER AND SIDE DISHES

Ham with Pineapple

Serves: 4

2 6-ounce ham steaks
3 tablespoons sugar-free maple syrup
4 slices canned pineapple in its own
    juice

Place ham steaks in an 8-inch baking pan. Cover with maple syrup. Arrange 2 pineapple slices on each steak. Bake at 450 degrees for approximately 20 minutes. Slice steaks in half to serve.

NUTRITIONAL ANALYSIS PER SERVING				
	Calories	118	Fiber	0 g
	Carbohydrates	10 g	Protein	14 g
	Sugar	7 g	Calcium	11 mg
	Total Fat	2.9 g	Vitamin A	18 I.U.
	Saturated Fat	1 g	Vitamin C	4 mg
	Cholesterol	45 mg	Folate	2 mcg
	Sodium	580 mg		

Veal Marsala

Serves: 2

6 ounces boneless veal steaks, cut very
    thin (¼ inch or less)
¼ cup egg substitute
¼ cup whole-wheat flour

½ cup Marsala cooking wine
1½ cups fresh sliced mushrooms
1 teaspoon minced onion
¼ teaspoon NoSalt® (salt substitute)
¼ teaspoon freshly ground pepper

Dip veal in egg substitute. Coat with flour. Place in saucepan well coated with cooking spray. Cook on high until golden on both sides. Reduce heat. Add wine, mushrooms, onion, and seasonings. Cover and cook until mushrooms are tender and sauce has reduced and thickened.

NUTRITIONAL ANALYSIS PER SERVING					
	Calories	206	Fiber	2 g
	Carbohydrates	14 g	Protein	20 g
	Sugar	4 g	Calcium	34 mg
	Total Fat	3.2 g	Vitamin A	77 I.U.
	Saturated Fat	0.8 g	Vitamin C	1 mg
	Cholesterol	65 mg	Folate	21 mcg
	Sodium	80 mg		

Crispy Chicken Dijon

Great for the kids!

Serves: 5

6 ounces plain fat-free yogurt
¼ cup honey Dijon mustard
2 packets Sweet'n Low®
10 1.5-ounce skinless chicken breast
    tenders
1 cup crushed low-fat or fat-free
    potato chips (Pringles® or similar)
Nonstick butter-flavored cooking
    spray

Combine yogurt, mustard, and Sweet'n Low®. Coat chicken breast tenders with the mixture. Top with crushed potato chips. Arrange in 13-by-9-inch pan sprayed well with cooking spray. Bake at 400 degrees for approximately 30 minutes.

NUTRITIONAL ANALYSIS PER SERVING	Calories	195	Fiber	0.9 g
	Carbohydrates	18 g	Protein	22 g
	Sugar	9 g	Calcium	73 mg
	Total Fat	3.9 g	Vitamin A	167 I.U.
	Saturated Fat	0.6 g	Vitamin C	3 mg
	Cholesterol	50 mg	Folate	4 mcg
	Sodium	165 mg		

Tomato Chevre Salad

B

Serves: 1

1 medium tomato, sliced
1 ounce chevre (goat cheese)
1 tablespoon red wine vinegar
1 teaspoon olive oil
Fresh basil, NoSalt® (salt substitute),
    and pepper to taste

Place tomato in small salad bowl. Arrange small cubes of cheese on top. Mix vinegar and oil and drizzle over salad. Garnish with basil and seasonings.

NUTRITIONAL ANALYSIS PER SERVING	Calories	143	Fiber	2 g
	Carbohydrates	6 g	Protein	7 g
	Sugar	4 g	Calcium	55 mg
	Total Fat	10.8 g	Vitamin A	1,534 I.U.
	Saturated Fat	4.8 g	Vitamin C	19 mg
	Cholesterol	13 mg	Folate	26 mcg
	Sodium	113 mg		

Nantucket Diet Wedge Salad

Serves: 4

1 whole head iceberg lettuce
2 cups chopped tomatoes
4 tablespoons imitation bacon bits
8 tablespoons Walden Farms® calorie-
    free blue cheese dressing

Slice head of lettuce into 4 quarters. Top each quarter with ½ cup tomatoes, 1 tablespoon bacon bits, and 2 tablespoons dressing.

NUTRITIONAL ANALYSIS PER SERVING	Calories	58	Fiber	2 g
	Carbohydrates	7 g	Protein	4 g
	Sugar	2 g	Calcium	32 mg
	Total Fat	2.1 g	Vitamin A	1,011 I.U.
	Saturated Fat	0.3 g	Vitamin C	15 mg
	Cholesterol	0 mg	Folate	68 mcg
	Sodium	406 mg		

Grilled Onions and Peppers

 Serves: 2

½ cup sliced onions
½ cup sliced green peppers
¼ cup low-sodium beef or vegetable
   broth
1 tablespoon squeezable nonfat margarine
½ tablespoon Mrs. Dash® Grilling
   Blends for beef

Place all ingredients in a small skillet. Cook until onions and peppers have browned and broth has reduced. Serve on top of grilled or broiled steak.

NUTRITIONAL ANALYSIS PER SERVING				
Calories	21	Fiber	1 g
Carbohydrates	5 g	Protein	1 g
Sugar	2 g	Calcium	9 mg
Total Fat	0.1 g	Vitamin A	86 I.U.
Saturated Fat	0 g	Vitamin C	20 mg
Cholesterol	0 mg	Folate	8 mcg
Sodium	62 mg		

DESSERT

Vanilla Chip Brownie Cake

 Serves: 16

3 ounces semisweet chocolate
½ cup Promise® Ultra Light margarine
1 cup Splenda®
3 tablespoons sugar
2 eggs
¾ cup all-purpose flour
1½ teaspoons baking powder
¼ cup vanilla baking chips

Place chocolate and margarine in a small bowl in the microwave and heat until melted, approximately 3 minutes. Beat Splenda®, sugar, and eggs until fluffy. Add flour, baking powder, and melted chocolate and margarine. Mix well. Stir in vanilla chips. Place in an 8-inch square pan coated well with nonstick cooking spray. Bake at 350 degrees for about 25 minutes.

NUTRITIONAL ANALYSIS PER SERVING				
Calories	114	Fiber	0 g
Carbohydrates	16 g	Protein	2 g
Sugar	10 g	Calcium	51 mg
Total Fat	4.4 g	Vitamin A	281 I.U.
Saturated Fat	2.4 g	Vitamin C	0 mg
Cholesterol	27 mg	Folate	14 mcg
Sodium	116 mg		

Sugar-Free Rocky Road Ice Cream Sandwich

Serves: 1

2 sugar-free Archway® soft rocky road
  cookies
3 tablespoons fat-free or low-fat
  sugar-free vanilla ice cream

Place ice cream on the flat side of one cookie and top it with the other
cookie. You can make several of them ahead, wrap them in plastic wrap,
and store them in the freezer. They are a fast frozen treat.
Variation: Try sugar-free chocolate chip, sugar, or peanut butter cookies.
You can also experiment with different ice cream flavors.

NUTRITIONAL ANALYSIS PER SERVING				
Calories	243	Fiber	2 g
Carbohydrates	38 g	Protein	4 g
Sugar	7 g	Calcium	118 mg
Total Fat	10.6 g	Vitamin A	119 I.U.
Saturated Fat	2.7 g	Vitamin C	0 mg
Cholesterol	2 mg	Folate	26 mcg
Sodium	150 mg		

Quick Key Lime Pie

Serves: 8

1 packaged low-fat graham cracker
  crust
1 envelope (¼ ounce) unflavored
  gelatin
1¾ cups low-fat (1%) milk
1 package (12 ounces) light (reduced-
  fat) cream cheese, softened
½ cup fresh lime juice
½ cup plus 2 tablespoons Splenda®
Lime slices and raspberries (optional)

Sprinkle gelatin over ½ cup milk in small saucepan; let stand 2 to 3 minutes. Add 2 tablespoons Splenda®. Cook over low heat, stirring constantly until gelatin is dissolved. Beat cream cheese in small bowl until fluffy; beat in remaining 1¼ cups milk and gelatin mixture. Mix in lime juice and ½ cup Splenda®. Fold into prepared crust and refrigerate pie until set, about 2 hours. Garnish with lime slices and raspberries if desired.

NUTRITIONAL ANALYSIS PER SERVING				
Calories	220	Fiber	0 g
Carbohydrates	23 g	Protein	8 g
Sugar	9 g	Calcium	113 mg
Total Fat	10.7 g	Vitamin A	644 I.U.
Saturated Fat	5.5 g	Vitamin C	5 mg
Cholesterol	23 mg	Folate	4 mcg
Sodium	313 mg		

Chocolate Almond Cookies

 Serves: 16 (1 cookie per serving)

1 cup all-purpose flour
1 egg
¾ cup plus 1 tablespoon Splenda®
¼ cup plus 2 tablespoons Benecol® or
   light margarine
1 teaspoon almond extract
1 teaspoon vanilla extract
½ teaspoon baking powder
1½ tablespoons unsweetened cocoa
   powder
1 tablespoon confectioner's sugar

Combine flour, egg, ¾ cup Splenda®, margarine, almond and vanilla extracts, baking powder, and cocoa powder. Mix well. Using hands, shape dough into 16 1-inch balls. Place 2 inches apart on nonstick cookie sheet. Bake at 350 degrees for approximately 15 minutes. Mix confectioner's sugar and 1 tablespoon Splenda® together. When cookies are cool, sprinkle mixture on top of cookies.

NUTRITIONAL ANALYSIS PER SERVING				
Calories	73	Fiber	0 g
Carbohydrates	8 g	Protein	1 g
Sugar	1 g	Calcium	12 mg
Total Fat	3.8 g	Vitamin A	203 I.U.
Saturated Fat	.5 g	Vitamin C	0 mg
Cholesterol	13 mg	Folate	16 mcg
Sodium	61 mg		

Chocolate-Dipped Strawberries

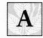

Serves: 12 (1 berry per serving)

12 large strawberries
2 ounces semisweet baking chocolate
    squares
Nonstick cooking spray

Remove stems from strawberries. Rinse and dry. Place chocolate squares in a cup or small bowl. Microwave for approximately 2 minutes, until melted. Dip ends of strawberries in chocolate and place on wax paper lightly coated with nonstick cooking spray. Chill and serve.
Variation: Try using white baking chocolate.

NUTRITIONAL ANALYSIS PER SERVING				
	Calories	32	Fiber	1 g
	Carbohydrates	5 g	Protein	0 g
	Sugar	4 g	Calcium	6 mg
	Total Fat	1.5 g	Vitamin A	3 I.U.
	Saturated Fat	0.8 g	Vitamin C	17 mg
	Cholesterol	0 mg	Folate	7 mcg
	Sodium	1 mg		

Nantucket Blueberry Shortcake

 Serves: 4

4 premade dessert shells (found in
   supermarket bakery or produce
   area)
1 package fat-free, sugar-free vanilla
   pudding mix
2 cups skim milk
2 cups fresh blueberries
1 tablespoon vanilla extract
4 packets sugar substitute
8 tablespoons fat-free frozen whipped
   topping

In a bowl, marinate blueberries with sugar substitute and vanilla. Follow
package directions for pudding. Top each dessert shell with one chilled
serving of vanilla pudding. Pour ½ cup blueberries over pudding and
garnish with 2 tablespoons whipped topping.

NUTRITIONAL ANALYSIS PER SERVING				
	Calories	190	Fiber	2 g
	Carbohydrates	30 g	Protein	6 g
	Sugar	20 g	Calcium	136 mg
	Total Fat	1.1 g	Vitamin A	334 I.U.
	Saturated Fat	0.3 g	Vitamin C	7 mg
	Cholesterol	31 mg	Folate	24 mcg
	Sodium	129 mg		

HEALTHY SNACKS:
DRINKS AND SMOOTHIES

Chocolate Frost

Serves: 1

½ cup skim milk
½ cup water
1 packet Swiss Miss®
    Diet Hot Chocolate
4 packets artificial sweetener
1 cup ice cubes

Place milk, water, hot chocolate, and sweetener packets in a blender. Add ice cubes. Blend until smooth and creamy.

Variations: Add 1 heaping teaspoon instant coffee for Mocha Frost or 1 scoop protein powder for Chocolate Protein Shake. Protein powder will add approximately 50–80 calories.

NUTRITIONAL ANALYSIS PER SERVING				
Calories	83	Fiber	0 g
Carbohydrates	14 g	Protein	6 g
Sugar	5 g	Calcium	111 mg
Total Fat	0.1 g	Vitamin A	250 I.U.
Saturated Fat	0.1 g	Vitamin C	0 mg
Cholesterol	2 mg	Folate	6 mcg
Sodium	204 mg		

Banana Strawberry Smoothie

B

Serves: 1

¼ cup water
1 6-ounce container light nonfat
    strawberry-banana yogurt
½ banana
4 packets artificial sweetener
1 cup ice cubes

Place water, yogurt, banana, and artificial sweetener in blender. Add ice cubes. Blend until smooth and creamy.
Variation: Add one packet of Benefiber® (all-natural fiber). Adds 20 calories to recipe and gives a fiber boost.

NUTRITIONAL ANALYSIS PER SERVING				
Calories	151	Fiber	1 g
Carbohydrates	32 g	Protein	7 g
Sugar	22 g	Calcium	265 mg
Total Fat	0.2 g	Vitamin A	32 I.U.
Saturated Fat	0.1 g	Vitamin C	8 mg
Cholesterol	4 mg	Folate	10 mcg
Sodium	105 mg		

Blueberry Tofu Smoothie

B

Serves: 1

¼ cup water
⅓ cup skim milk
¼ container light tofu (113 grams)

½ teaspoon vanilla extract
⅓ cup fresh blueberries
3–4 packets Sweet'n Low®
1 cup ice cubes

Place all ingredients in blender. Blend until smooth and creamy.

NUTRITIONAL ANALYSIS PER SERVING	Calories	112	Fiber	1 g
	Carbohydrates	15 g	Protein	10 g
	Sugar	8 g	Calcium	118 mg
	Total Fat	1.1 g	Vitamin A	193 I.U.
	Saturated Fat	0.2 g	Vitamin C	5 mg
	Cholesterol	2 mg	Folate	7 mcg
	Sodium	133 mg		

Vanilla Soy Yogurt Smoothie

Serves: 1

¾ cup vanilla soy milk
1 6-ounce container fat-free vanilla
    yogurt
1½ teaspoons vanilla extract
3–4 packets Sweet'n Low®
1 cup ice cubes

Place soy milk, yogurt, vanilla extract, and sweetener in blender. Add ice cubes. Blend until smooth and creamy.
Variation: For Chocolate Soy Yogurt Smoothie, use chocolate soy milk and add 1 tablespoon sugar-free chocolate syrup (adds 10 calories).

NUTRITIONAL ANALYSIS PER SERVING	Calories	143	Fiber	0 g
	Carbohydrates	18 g	Protein	8 g
	Sugar	14 g	Calcium	225 mg
	Total Fat	0 g	Vitamin A	749 I.U.
	Saturated Fat	0 g	Vitamin C	9 mg
	Cholesterol	4 mg	Folate	0 mcg
	Sodium	101 mg		

Coffee Frost

Serves: 1

1 teaspoon instant coffee
½ cup skim milk
½ cup water
1 cup ice cubes
3–4 packets artificial sweetener

Place all ingredients in a blender. Blend until smooth and creamy.

NUTRITIONAL ANALYSIS PER SERVING	Calories	56	Fiber	0 g
	Carbohydrates	9 g	Protein	4 g
	Sugar	3 g	Calcium	113 mg
	Total Fat	0.1 g	Vitamin A	250 I.U.
	Saturated Fat	0.1 g	Vitamin C	0 mg
	Cholesterol	2 mg	Folate	6 mcg
	Sodium	54 mg		

Tropical Tofu Shake

Serves: 1

6 ounces pineapple juice
¼ package light tofu (99 grams)
¼ cup sliced banana
2 teaspoons coconut extract
3 packages artificial sweetener
1 cup ice cubes

Place pineapple juice, tofu, banana, coconut extract, sweetener, and ice cubes into blender. Blend until smooth and creamy.

NUTRITIONAL ANALYSIS PER SERVING					
Calories	222		Fiber	1 g
Carbohydrates	36 g		Protein	7 g
Sugar	31 g		Calcium	66 mg
Total Fat	1.1 g		Vitamin A	33 I.U.
Saturated Fat	0.2 g		Vitamin C	21 mg
Cholesterol	0 mg		Folate	47 mcg
Sodium	86 mg			

LIGHT BITES

Cheese Popcorn

Serves: 1

4 cups air-popped popcorn, no salt
   added
2 tablespoons parmesan

Place popcorn in a bowl and top with cheese. Serve immediately. Popcorn is best when warm.

NUTRITIONAL ANALYSIS PER SERVING	Calories	165	Fiber	5 g
	Carbohydrates	25 g	Protein	5 g
	Sugar	0 g	Calcium	66 mg
	Total Fat	4.2 g	Vitamin A	107 I.U.
	Saturated Fat	1.9 g	Vitamin C	0 mg
	Cholesterol	9 mg	Folate	8 mcg
	Sodium	154 mg		

Sweet Cinnamon Popcorn

B *Serves:* 1

4 cups air-popped popcorn, no salt
    added
½ tablespoon Splenda®
⅛ teaspoon cinnamon

Mix Splenda® and cinnamon together. Sprinkle over popcorn.

NUTRITIONAL ANALYSIS PER SERVING	Calories	130	Fiber	4 g
	Carbohydrates	21 g	Protein	3 g
	Sugar	0 g	Calcium	8 mg
	Total Fat	1 g	Vitamin A	65 I.U.
	Saturated Fat	0.1 g	Vitamin C	0 mg
	Cholesterol	0 mg	Folate	6 mcg
	Sodium	1 mg		

Chicken Tacos

 B

Serves: 10

1 pound ground chicken
1 package low-sodium taco seasoning
   mix
⅔ cup water
10 yellow corn taco shells
10 tablespoons reduced-fat Mexican
   or taco blend shredded cheese
10 tablespoons shredded lettuce
2 tomatoes, diced

Place chicken in skillet, separate into small pieces, and brown on all sides. Add seasoning and water; simmer until sauce thickens. Place taco shells in the oven at 350 degrees for 3 minutes, until warm. Fill shells with ground chicken (about 1.5 ounces per taco). Top each shell with 1 tablespoon cheese, approximately 2 tablespoons lettuce, and 1 tablespoon tomato.

NUTRITIONAL ANALYSIS PER SERVING				
	Calories	170	Fiber	1 g
	Carbohydrates	13 g	Protein	10 g
	Sugar	1 g	Calcium	89 mg
	Total Fat	8.2 g	Vitamin A	429 I.U.
	Saturated Fat	2.2 g	Vitamin C	4 mg
	Cholesterol	35 mg	Folate	5 mcg
	Sodium	429 mg		

Veggie Pocket Sandwich

Serves: 1

1 mini whole-wheat pita bread
2 tablespoons alfalfa sprouts
1 tablespoon shredded carrots
2 tomato slices
3 cucumber slices
3 green pepper slices
1 tablespoon grated parmesan cheese
1 tablespoon fat-free ranch dressing

Slice top of pita. Place all ingredients inside and serve.

NUTRITIONAL ANALYSIS PER SERVING				
	Calories	110	Fiber	3 g
	Carbohydrates	19 g	Protein	5 g
	Sugar	2 g	Calcium	70 mg
	Total Fat	2.3 g	Vitamin A	1,664 I.U.
	Saturated Fat	1.0 g	Vitamin C	14 mg
	Cholesterol	4 mg	Folate	22 mcg
	Sodium	368 mg		

Veggie Pita Pizza

Serves: 6

6 whole-wheat mini pita breads
12 tablespoons Healthy Choice®
   Roasted Garlic Primavera
   tomato sauce
6 tablespoons chopped green
   pepper pieces
24 slices mushroom

9 tablespoons Italian-style five-cheese
shredded cheese

Place foil on baking sheet. Arrange pita breads on foil. Place 2 tablespoons
sauce on each bread. Top each pita with 1 tablespoon green pepper and 4
mushroom slices. Sprinkle each pita with 1½ tablespoons cheese. Bake at
350 degrees for 20–25 minutes or until the cheese is golden brown.

NUTRITIONAL ANALYSIS PER SERVING	Calories	115	Fiber	1 g
	Carbohydrates	18 g	Protein	5 g
	Sugar	2 g	Calcium	70 mg
	Total Fat	3 g	Vitamin A	276 I.U.
	Saturated Fat	1.5 g	Vitamin C	9 mg
	Cholesterol	7 mg	Folate	11 mcg
	Sodium	296 mg		

Zesty Tomato Tofu Dip

Serves: 8 (2 tablespoons per serving)

¼ container light tofu (113 grams)
6 tablespoons light sour cream
¼ cup tomato juice
1 teaspoon Worcestershire sauce
1 tablespoon low-salt ketchup
2 packets Sweet'n Low®
Dash celery salt

Place all ingredients in a bowl; beat with electric mixer until smooth.

NUTRITIONAL ANALYSIS PER SERVING	Calories	23	Fiber	0 g
	Carbohydrates	3 g	Protein	1 g
	Sugar	2 g	Calcium	22 mg
	Total Fat	0.9 g	Vitamin A	126 I.U.
	Saturated Fat	0.6 g	Vitamin C	1 mg
	Cholesterol	4 mg	Folate	0 mcg
	Sodium	65 mg		

Holiday Cheer

Cranberry Walnut Salad with Cranberry Vinaigrette

Serves: 1

3 cups lettuce
2 tablespoons dried cranberries
1 tablespoon chopped walnuts
½ cup light cranberry juice
½ tablespoon cornstarch
1 tablespoon red wine vinegar
2 packets artificial sweetener

Place lettuce, cranberries, and walnuts in a bowl. Toss. Place remaining ingredients in a cup or small bowl. Mix well. Microwave on high until mixture begins to boil. Mix well again. Vinaigrette should start to thicken. Chill. Use 2 tablespoons dressing for salad and reserve the rest for another use.

NUTRITIONAL ANALYSIS PER SERVING				
Calories	123	Fiber	3 g
Carbohydrates	19 g	Protein	3 g
Sugar	13 g	Calcium	65 mg
Total Fat	5.3 g	Vitamin A	5,466 I.U.
Saturated Fat	0.5 g	Vitamin C	6 mg
Cholesterol	0 mg	Folate	128 mcg
Sodium	9 mg		

Sweet Winter Squash

Serves: 2

1½ cups fresh or frozen winter squash
2 tablespoons squeezable nonfat mar-
    garine
1½ tablespoons imitation brown sugar
    (Sugar Twin® or similar)

Prepare squash: chop, boil, and mash for fresh, or microwave for frozen.
Mix in margarine and imitation brown sugar and serve.

NUTRITIONAL ANALYSIS PER SERVING				
Calories	71	Fiber	5 g
Carbohydrates	18 g	Protein	1 g
Sugar	1 g	Calcium	57 mg
Total Fat	0.2 g	Vitamin A	1,501 I.U.
Saturated Fat	0 g	Vitamin C	12 mg
Cholesterol	0 mg	Folate	20 mcg
Sodium	21 mg		

Glazed Carrots

Serves: 2

1 pound fresh whole baby carrots
¼ cup sugar-free maple syrup
2 tablespoons squeezable nonfat mar-
    garine
Dash ginger
1–2 packets artificial sweetener
    (optional)

Boil or steam carrots until tender. Drain and add syrup, margarine, ginger, and sweetener. Mix and serve.

NUTRITIONAL ANALYSIS PER SERVING				
Calories	87	Fiber	4 g
Carbohydrates	19 g	Protein	1 g
Sugar	11 g	Calcium	73 mg
Total Fat	0.3 g	Vitamin A	31,776 I.U.
Saturated Fat	0.1 g	Vitamin C	19 g
Cholesterol	0 mg	Folate	75 mcg
Sodium	279 mg		

Kay's Stuffing

Serves: 12

1 15-ounce package country-style sea-
    soned stuffing cubes
2 sticks (1 cup) margarine
1 cup chopped onion

1 cup chopped celery
1½–2 teaspoons Bell's® Seasoning
Half a reduced-fat pork sausage
   (6 ounces)
2 cups fat-free, reduced-sodium
   chicken broth
Dash pepper
¼ teaspoon salt

In saucepan, melt margarine; add onion, celery, Bell's® seasoning, salt, and pepper. Sauté until onion and celery are softened. In separate saucepan, cook sausage until brown. Add the cooked sausage to the vegetable mixture. Place seasoned stuffing in a large mixing bowl. Heat the chicken broth in the microwave until hot. Add vegetable mixture and chicken broth to the seasoned stuffing cubes. Fork mixture and cubes together. Cover and let stand for 5–10 minutes. Stuffs a 14-to-18-pound turkey.

If you prefer more of a sausage taste, then add three-quarters or the whole sausage. You can also substitute cubes of light white and/or wheat bread for the packaged stuffing.

NUTRITIONAL ANALYSIS PER SERVING				
	Calories	260	Fiber	3 g
	Carbohydrates	29 g	Protein	5 g
	Sugar	3 g	Calcium	40 mg
	Total Fat	13.4 g	Vitamin A	720 I.U.
	Saturated Fat	1.4 g	Vitamin C	1 mg
	Cholesterol	1 mg	Folate	5 mcg
	Sodium	822 mg		

Grandma Coffin's Cranberry Crumble

Serves: 9

1 cup rolled oats
1 cup light brown sugar
½ cup flour
1 stick (½ cup) margarine
1 16-ounce can whole cranberry sauce

Place oats, brown sugar, and flour in a bowl. Melt the margarine and add it to dry ingredients. Mix until crumbly. Spray 8-inch pan with non-stick cooking spray. Press half of oat mixture into pan. Cover with cranberry sauce. Sprinkle remaining oat mixture over the top. Bake at 350 degrees for 30 minutes.

NUTRITIONAL ANALYSIS PER SERVING				
Calories	290	Fiber	2 g
Carbohydrates	53 g	Protein	2 g
Sugar	35 g	Calcium	26 mg
Total Fat	8.6 g	Vitamin A	453 I.U.
Saturated Fat	1 g	Vitamin C	0 mg
Cholesterol	0 mg	Folate	14 mcg
Sodium	118 mg		

Sandy's Pumpkin Maple Pie

Serves: 10

1⅓ cups all-purpose flour
½ cup plus 1 tablespoon Splenda®

¾ teaspoon Salt Sense® (33% less
  sodium)
3 tablespoons vegetable shortening
2 tablespoons margarine
4 to 5 tablespoons ice water
1 15-ounce can solid pack pumpkin
2 egg whites
1 cup evaporated skim milk
⅓ cup sugar-free maple syrup
½ teaspoon cinnamon
½ teaspoon ginger
2 tablespoons brown sugar
Light or fat-free whipped topping
  (optional)

Combine flour, 1 tablespoon Splenda®, and ¼ teaspoon Salt Sense® in medium bowl. Mix in shortening and margarine until mixture looks like crumbs. Mix in ice water, 1 tablespoon at a time, until mixture comes together and forms a soft dough. Wrap in plastic and refrigerate 30 minutes. Preheat oven to 425 degrees. Roll out pastry on floured surface to ⅛-inch thickness. Cut into circle and place into 9-inch pie plate. Turn edges under and flute. Combine pumpkin, remaining ½ cup Splenda®, egg whites, milk, maple syrup, cinnamon, ginger, brown sugar, and remaining ½ teaspoon Salt Sense® in large bowl. Mix well. Pour into unbaked pie shell. Bake 15 minutes. Reduce oven temperature to 350 degrees. Continue baking until center is set, 45 to 50 minutes. Transfer to wire rack. Let stand 30 minutes before serving. Garnish each serving with 2 tablespoons whipped topping, if desired.

NUTRITIONAL ANALYSIS PER SERVING	Calories	187	Fiber	2 g
	Carbohydrates	27 g	Protein	5 g
	Sugar	8 g	Calcium	92 mg
	Total Fat	6.8 g	Vitamin A	6,820 I.U.
	Saturated Fat	2.2 g	Vitamin C	2 mg
	Cholesterol	1 mg	Folate	38 mcg
	Sodium	161 mg		

NANTUCKET DIET COCKTAILS

Nantucket D'Light

Serves: 1

2.5 ounces Triple Eight vodka™
   (product of Nantucket)
3 ounces sparkling water or calorie-
   free soda
Splash of light cranberry juice
1 lime wedge
Ice

Place ice in cocktail glass. Add vodka, soda, and cranberry juice and garnish with lime.

NUTRITIONAL ANALYSIS PER SERVING					
Calories	173		Fiber	0 g	
Carbohydrates	2 g		Protein	0 g	
Sugar	2 g		Calcium	0 mg	
Total Fat	0 g		Vitamin A	1 I.U.	
Saturated Fat	0 mg		Vitamin C	6 mg	
Cholesterol	0 g		Folate	0 mcg	
Sodium	0 mg				

Nantucket Diet Red

Serves: 1

2.5 ounces Triple Eight vodka™
4 ounces diet raspberry ginger ale
Ice

Place ice in cocktail glass. Add vodka and ginger ale.

NUTRITIONAL ANALYSIS PER SERVING				
Calories	164	Fiber	0 g
Carbohydrates	0 g	Protein	0 g
Sugar	0 g	Calcium	0 mg
Total Fat	0 g	Vitamin A	0 I.U.
Saturated Fat	0 g	Vitamin C	0 mg
Cholesterol	0 mg	Folate	0 mcg
Sodium	24 mg		

Nantucket Diet Hurricane

B

Serves: 1

2.5 ounces Hurricane rum
(product of Nantucket)
4 ounces diet cola
1 lemon wedge
Ice

Place ice in tall cocktail glass. Add rum and diet cola. Garnish with lemon.

NUTRITIONAL ANALYSIS PER SERVING				
Calories	165	Fiber	0 g
Carbohydrates	0 g	Protein	0 g
Sugar	0 g	Calcium	3 g
Total Fat	0 g	Vitamin A	0 I.U.
Saturated Fat	0 g	Vitamin C	0 mg
Cholesterol	0 mg	Folate	0 mcg
Sodium	6 mg		

Special Events

ENJOY NANTUCKET

Enjoy Nantucket is a catering company owned and operated by Ben Goldberg. The inspiration for the company began years ago, when he began to cook, and feed his friends and family. As he grew older, he became more adventurous in his culinary explorations. His career started with a love of entertaining and making people happy the best way he knew how—through their taste buds and bellies. This love has continued in his ventures on Nantucket.

Goldberg's dishes are fresh, healthy, and very Nantucket. To support the local merchants (without whom much of the flavor in his dishes would be impossible), he likes to use products from local bakeries, farms, and specialty shops. His dishes are simple but tasty, and the flavors and recipes are clear and delicious.

Great Point is one of the best places in the world to have a barbecue. To get to Great Point, on the easternmost point of the island, you will need a car, a tire pressure gauge, and a permit to drive on the beach. But the breathtaking views are well worth the trouble: you will never see a more beautiful sunset. The vistas are only enhanced by these simple, fun, and delicious recipes.

A Great Point BBQ

ITEMS TO BRING TO A GREAT POINT BARBECUE

REQUIRED

Air pump and tire pressure gauge (to drive on the soft sand, tire pressure must be reduced to 12 psi)

2 Weber charcoal grills

Match Light charcoal

Lighter or matches

Metal tongs

Metal spatula

Sharp knife

Large cutting board

Paper plates

Napkins

Trash bags

Small folding table

2 coolers (fill the first cooler with 2 bottles of wine, some bottles of beer, and Nantucket Nectars juices, fresh drinking water, and soda; the second cooler should be for food only)

OPTIONAL

Silverware

Premoistened towelettes

Beach chairs

Blankets

Fishing poles

Frisbee

Football

Beach tennis set

Tiki torches

Beef Teriyaki Skewers

This item is a kids' favorite, but it has a sophisticated flavor that adults love too. You can marinate these for at least a day ahead of time (a few hours will also infuse the beef with plenty of flavor). Once again, the only work to do at the beach is the grilling.

Serves: 20 (1 skewer per serving)

8 ounces soy sauce
8 ounces brown sugar

2 tablespoons fresh chopped garlic
2 tablespoons fresh grated ginger
1 teaspoon hot red pepper flakes
3 pounds sirloin tips, sliced into 1-inch
     strips
20 wooden skewers (soak in water
     overnight to prevent burning)

Whisk together soy sauce, brown sugar, garlic, ginger, and red pepper flakes. Add beef and marinate for up to 2 days. Thread beef tips onto skewers.

Place beef skewers on grill and cook 4 minutes per side (or to order). Serve hot off the grill to the nearest person.

NUTRITIONAL ANALYSIS PER SERVING	Calories	105	Fiber	0 g
	Carbohydrates	3 g	Protein	14 g
	Sugar	3 g	Calcium	7 mg
	Total Fat	3.8 g	Vitamin A	15 I.U.
	Saturated Fat	1.4 g	Vitamin C	0 mg
	Cholesterol	44 mg	Folate	5 mcg
	Sodium	177 mg		

Seawater Corn on the Cob

Late August is the best time to get delicious, fresh sweet corn on Nantucket. Any variety will do, as long as the kernels are plump and the husk intact. I like to steam corn in the husk for two reasons: the flavors of the corn (when steamed in its own greens) are enhanced, and the peeled-back husk makes for a great handle. Corn is best eaten al dente—try not to overcook it. It is tasty and healthy eaten plain because the seawater will infuse this sweet vegetable with a salty flavor.

Serves: 10

10 ears corn in the husk
Seawater

Gather your "sous chefs" to submerge the ears of corn, in the husk, in the ocean. Place up to ten ears of corn at a time on the grill; cover. Rotate corn periodically, until the green husks are slightly burnt. Depending on your fire, this can take anywhere from 10 to 12 minutes. Remove corn from the grill and let cool for 5 minutes. Peel back the husk from the corn and eat.

NUTRITIONAL ANALYSIS PER SERVING	Calories	80	Fiber	3 g
	Carbohydrates	18 g	Protein	3 g
	Sugar	5 g	Calcium	0 mg
	Total Fat	1 g	Vitamin A	100 I.U.
	Saturated Fat	0 g	Vitamin C	6 mg
	Cholesterol	0 mg	Folate	0 mcg
	Sodium	0 mg		

By now, the sun should be setting off shore. This is a good time to take some casts with a fishing rod: bluefish and striped bass run close to the tip of the point around sunset. If you are lucky, the moon will rise over the lighthouse while the sun goes down over the ocean. At this point, you can either gather all your guests, clean up, and head back home, or stay out and gaze at the starry night sky. Family, friends, great food, and the beauty of this one-of-a-kind culinary sunset adventure make for an unforgettable experience.

A Light Luncheon

Goldberg loves preparing healthy, delicious luncheons. The following recipes are simple, and the best part is that most of these flavors expand over time; in other words, you can prepare these dishes in the morning (or even the night before), and the resulting tastes will be strong and vibrant.

As a caterer, the most problems in the kitchen arise during last-minute cooking. These recipes minimize the amount of time spent on last-minute cooking, which guarantees a smoother and more enjoyable experience for both host and guest. *Do not be afraid to use some store-bought prepared items to save time.*

The idea of a light Nantucket luncheon involves basic, high-flavor, low-calorie foods. Some tips: use fresh, summery ingredients, flavor with fresh lemon juice, and substitute different mustards for mayonnaise. Variety is also of the utmost importance, not only to satisfy the varied tastes of your guests (while promoting a certain continuity of flavor) but also because different diets restrict different foods.

Goldberg firmly believes that every meal needs to be finished with something sweet to keep the luncheon light and simple (yet satisfying). He puts together a platter with different small fresh-baked desserts from the many bakeries around the island. This allows the individual guest to choose how to satisfy his or her sweet tooth in a small portion. The quantities in this menu allow for leftovers: it is great to give the guests something to go home with.

My Lobster Rolls

If you are having a lobster dinner, Goldberg suggests always ordering extra to make sure you have enough to make this lobster salad. The flavor should come from the fresh lemon juice, not the mayonnaise. These taste great on toasted hot dog buns.

Serves: 15

2 pounds fresh lobster meat, cooked
2 lemons
1 teaspoon sea salt
½ teaspoon freshly ground pepper
1 cup sliced celery
½ cup diced sweet onion (Vidalia or
    Spanish)
¼ cup mayonnaise
1 teaspoon Dijon mustard
½ teaspoon hot pepper sauce
    (optional)
15 hot dog buns

Making sure all the shells are removed, roughly chop the lobster meat. Squeeze the juice of the lemons on the lobster meat; season with salt and pepper. Mix in the celery and onions with your clean hands or a spoon. Fold in the mayonnaise and the mustard (and hot pepper sauce, if desired). This mixture will keep, covered and refrigerated, for up to three days. Fill warm, toasted hot dog buns with lobster salad just before the guests arrive. A real crowd-pleaser!

NUTRITIONAL ANALYSIS PER SERVING	Calories	210	Fiber	1 g
	Carbohydrates	23 g	Protein	17 g
	Sugar	3 g	Calcium	101 mg
	Total Fat	5.2 g	Vitamin A	96 I.U.
	Saturated Fat	0.9 g	Vitamin C	4 mg
	Cholesterol	45 mg	Folate	58 mcg
	Sodium	625 mg		

Grilled Pork Tenderloin with Fresh Peach Salsa

Summer on Nantucket, with its variety of fresh fruits, allows you to be creative with this dish. Pork tenderloin is very lean and can be served at room temperature with the fresh fruit salsa. You can grill the meat ahead of time and thinly slice just minutes before serving. You can replace the peaches with the freshest fruit available: mangoes and pineapple work very well, or you can even use other fruit such as cantaloupe or strawberries. Make the salsa up to 1 day ahead of time. The longer it sits, the better it will taste.

B *Serves: 15*

2 small peaches, diced (about 1 cup)
1 pint grape tomatoes, halved
½ cup diced red onion
¼ cup chopped fresh cilantro

2 tablespoons chopped jalapeño pepper (remove the seeds)

½ cup fresh corn, steamed and
removed from cob

2 cloves chopped fresh garlic (about
1 tablespoon)

¼ cup lime juice

¼ cup red wine vinegar

1 teaspoon kosher salt

Freshly ground pepper

4 pounds pork tenderloin (about 15
4-ounce pieces)

1 tablespoon olive oil

Mix all ingredients except pork together and let sit for at least 1 hour or overnight. Trim any fat from the pork tenderloin. Season with additional salt and pepper and rub with olive oil. Grill until tender. The temperature inside the thickest part of the meat must reach 140°—use a meat thermometer to measure. Let cool and slice thinly. Serve slices with cold or room-temperature peach salsa.

NUTRITIONAL ANALYSIS PER SERVING				
	Calories	168	Fiber	0 g
	Carbohydrates	5 g	Protein	26 g
	Sugar	1 g	Calcium	10 mg
	Total Fat	4.6 g	Vitamin A	195 I.U.
	Saturated Fat	1.5 g	Vitamin C	9 mg
	Cholesterol	79 mg	Folate	14 mcg
	Sodium	189 mg		

BEN GOLDBERG'S PHILOSOPHY AND DINING TIPS

When most of you are on Nantucket, you are on vacation. Relax. The food served at my parties is fresh and healthy. That said, a good tip for trying to eat healthy at a catered event is to stay away from most of the fried foods. Portion control is also very important: if you want to try everything on the buffet, make sure you limit your portions. Eat light the day of a catered event. That way, you can splurge a little when you arrive, and you will have the appetite to try new and delicious dishes. Have fun, and enjoy the flavors of Nantucket!

NANTUCKET CLAMBAKE COMPANY *and* SUSAN M. WARNER CATERING

Nantucket Clambake Company and Susan M. Warner Catering have been creating wonderful food and memories on Nantucket for over eighteen years. As a full-service catering company, they are available to plan all aspects of your events, or to simply coordinate the fine details. Whether it is a casual New England clambake for family and friends, a corporate event, or an elegant wedding for three hundred, they will help you capture the magic that is Nantucket Island.

NANTUCKET CLAMBAKE COMPANY

Traditional New England Pit Clambake

A "Make Love to Life" Meal

Everyone knows that food tastes better when eaten outside. Enjoying a traditional New England pit clambake at the edge of the sea is the ultimate outdoor eating experience. The sights and sounds of the sea combined with those of the pit bake create a wonderful way to enjoy great food with family and friends.

The traditional New England pit clambake comes from the cooking processes of Native Americans who cooked seafood in large fire pits. Preparing the beach pit and fire in which the food is cooked is the most time-consuming and exhausting part of the whole process, but it is well worth it.

Serves: 20

FOOD

20 1¼-pound lobsters
10 pounds steamers, rinsed
10 pounds mussels, debearded
25–35 small white onions, peeled
25–35 small new potatoes, scrubbed

3 dozen ears of sweet corn with outside husks removed

Lemon wedges

Melted butter (optional)

EQUIPMENT

Town permit and fire permit (check
with town offices in your area)

Rockweed (soaked but drained before
set on pit; it can be ordered ahead
from a fish market)

12-by-14-foot canvas tarp (soak in salt
or fresh water)

Rocks (dry rocks conduct heat better)

Wire baskets (or cheesecloth) to cook
seafood

Iron rakes and shovels

Fire gloves, aprons, towels

Matches, newspapers, and kindling to
start fire

Hardwood pallets (8–10) or firewood

Galvanized garbage can for the hot
embers

Trash containers

Lots of trash bags

Sharp knife for assorted tasks

Food tongs

Small pot for melting butter

Lobster crackers and picks

Knives, forks, and napkins or paper
towels

Bowls or plates for serving food

Fresh water for rinsing food dropped
in sand

DIGGING THE PIT

A large beach pit about 4 by 6 feet and 2 feet deep is dug in beach sand
and outlined with rocks about the size of large grapefruits. One strong
person can dig a pit like this in 20 minutes.

HEATING THE ROCKS

Authentic pit clambakes cook when the moisture from the rockweed creates steam with the radiating heat of the rocks (rockweed with pods works best because the pods contain small pockets of water). Hardwood such as oak or ash is best to use for the main fire. One may also use hardwood pallets (the ones that make you groan when you lift them!). The heat and hot steam that rise from the rocks essentially create your oven. Therefore heating the rocks is the most important step in the cooking process.

Lay kindling in the center of the pit (shingles or two-by-fours are fine). Then lay two hardwood pallets on top of the kindling. Place enough rocks on top of the pallets to cover the surface of the pallets. Ignite the fire. As the wood burns, it is replaced with more wood. Move the hot coals around with a shovel to evenly heat rocks underneath. The pit should be tended in this way for 3–4 hours.

SETTING THE PIT

Time is of the essence in this process. You do not want to lose any more of the heat in the rocks than is necessary. Quickly remove all coals with a shovel into a galvanized garbage can. If you do not remove almost all the coals, the food will have a smoky taste. As soon as the rocks are free of embers, lay 5 inches of rockweed on top of the hot rocks as quickly as possible. Then lay lobsters in wire baskets on the rockweed. Steamer clams and mussels in their own baskets are placed on top. Wire baskets with onions and new potatoes are placed next, followed by ears of sweet corn in their husks. (Instead of using wire metal baskets, food can be layered directly on top of rockweed or placed in cheesecloth bags.) A soaking-wet heavy canvas tarp is laid on top to steam the feast. Make sure that the canvas does not touch the hot rocks and that no steam escapes around the edges.

REMOVING THE FOOD FROM THE PIT

The best way to prevent overcooking or undercooking is to very carefully pull back a corner of the tarp wearing fire gloves and pull out a lobster. If you were the one cooking the lobsters, go ahead and split a tail open and taste . . . you deserve it. A well-set pit will cook in 45–60 minutes, but it could take up to 30 minutes longer. The tarp is then removed in a big salty, steamy cloud. Everything is perfectly cooked and flavored with the wonderful taste of the sea.

CLEANING UP

Leaving the beach as you found it is the most important part of your pit bake. If you brought the rocks with you, make sure you take them back with you, along with any embers, wood, or any other flotsam and jetsam left over from your pit bake. If all of this seems to be too much work, just call the Nantucket Clambake Company and enjoy!

NUTRITIONAL ANALYSIS PER SERVING	Calories	731	Fiber	11 g
	Carbohydrates	90 g	Protein	76 g
	Sugar	14 g	Calcium	223 mg
	Total Fat	8.8 g	Vitamin A	871 I.U.
	Saturated Fat	1.3 g	Vitamin C	86 mg
	Cholesterol	191 mg	Folate	167 mcg
	Sodium	1,257 mg		

SUSAN WARNER CATERING COMPANY

Orange Sesame Asian Salad with Lobster

A terrific first course, or light summer lunch, this is a perfect recipe for using leftover lobster meat from a clambake. If you have eaten all the lobsters at your clambake, you can cook two 1¼-pound lobsters and pick the meat yourself or have your local fish market prepare the meat. You may opt to buy three lobster tails and serve ½ to each person.

 Serves: 6

Orange Sesame Dressing

Makes ¾ cup

3 medium Valencia oranges
3 tablespoons sesame oil
2 tablespoons sesame seeds, toasted
Salt and pepper to taste

Make dressing a day ahead. Peel oranges with a knife (making sure white rind is completely removed) and cut into segments. Brown sesame seeds in a dry skillet over medium heat until golden, approximately 2 minutes. Leave to cool. Put orange, sesame seeds, and sesame oil in a blender. Blend until smooth, about 10 seconds on high. Add salt and pepper to taste. Put dressing in screw-top jar and refrigerate overnight.

Asian Salad

4 ounces mesclun mixed greens
3 stalks bok choy, white portions only,
    cut in half lengthwise and then
    thinly sliced, (if you cannot find
    bok choy, you can use Chinese cel-
    ery or Napa cabbage)
1½ cups fresh bean sprouts, coarsely
    chopped
¾ cup (about 6) small radishes, sliced
    thinly
1 cup (about 5 ounces) snow peas,
    trimmed and blanched for 1 minute
    in boiling water, drained and cut
    into thirds
1 medium carrot, grated

3 oranges, segmented and chopped
  into bite-size pieces, save some aside
  to top salad
¾ pound cooked lobster meat, cut into
  bite-sized pieces (or ½ lobster tail
  per person)
1 cup Chinese fried noodles (found in
  the Chinese food section), or
  1 ounce vermicelli noodles broken
  into small pieces and fried in
  peanut oil until golden brown
  (4–5 seconds)

Divide mesclun greens among six plates. Toss bok choy, bean sprouts, radishes, snow peas, carrots, and orange pieces with enough dressing to lightly coat. Toss lobster meat with dressing in a separate bowl. Some dressing will be left over. Place tossed vegetable mixture on greens. Divide and arrange the lobster meat and orange segments on top of the salads. Top each salad with a cluster of noodles.

NUTRITIONAL ANALYSIS PER SERVING				
Calories	284	Fiber	6 g
Carbohydrates	26 g	Protein	17 g
Sugar	16 g	Calcium	148 mg
Total Fat	13.3 g	Vitamin A	4,472 I.U.
Saturated Fat	2.1 g	Vitamin C	104 mg
Cholesterol	41 mg	Folate	122 mcg
Sodium	251 mg		

AVEC PANACHE

Avec Panache was founded in 1983 in Aspen, Colorado, by James Martinsson, a premier French chef. Martinsson found his way to Nantucket, where he continues to be an instructor of the culinary arts, specializing in classic French cuisine for adults and the younger generation. He also hosts guided tours of France, providing individuals with a true culinary and cultural experience.

Crab Salad Martinique

A "Make Love to Life" Meal

F | *Serves:* 4

8 cups arugula
1 tablespoon Dijon mustard
3 tablespoons balsamic vinegar
4 tablespoons extra-virgin olive oil
¼ cup diced mango
½ cup diced red and yellow tomato
½ cup basil chiffonade (loosely
　chopped into long strips)
kernels of corn from 2 cobs
½ cup cooked and drained orzo
2 tablespoons olive oil
1 tablespoon butter
1 graffiti eggplant or extra-small egg-
　plant, sliced ⅛ inch thick
2 eggs
Juice from one lemon
¼ cup chopped parsley
2 tablespoons unsalted clarified butter
8 slices (very thin) smoked salmon
4 tablespoons light sour cream
16 ounces fresh crabmeat

Place the mustard in a bowl. Whisk in the vinegar and then drizzle in oil
while continuing to whisk. Toss arugula with vinaigrette.

Lightly sauté mango, tomato, basil, corn, and orzo with olive oil and
butter for 3–5 minutes.

Beat eggs. Dip sliced eggplant in eggs and sauté lightly.

Combine lemon juice, parsley, and butter. Use to top crabmeat.

Assemble on each plate 2 cups arugula, surrounded by salsa, top
with eggplant. Add 2 very thin slices smoked salmon, 1 tablespoon sour
cream, and 4 ounces crabmeat topped with the warm sauce.

NUTRITIONAL ANALYSIS PER SERVING	Calories	567	Fiber	3 g
	Carbohydrates	26 g	Protein	36 g
	Sugar	9 g	Calcium	244 mg
	Total Fat	36.6 g	Vitamin A	2,188 I.U.
	Saturated Fat	9.9 g	Vitamin C	31 mg
	Cholesterol	253 mg	Folate	147 mcg
	Sodium	1,022 mg		

French Onion Soup

Serves: 6

2 tablespoons unsalted butter
1 small red onion, thinly sliced
3 white onions, thinly sliced
1 clove garlic, finely chopped
3 tablespoons all-purpose flour (may
    omit for a lighter soup)
¾ cup white wine
6 cups brown stock (or water for a
    lighter soup)
Bouquet garni*
Salt
Pepper
1 tablespoon sherry
6 ½-inch-thick slices of French
    baguette
1½ cups finely grated Gruyère

Melt the butter in a large, heavy-bottomed saucepan over medium heat.
Add the onions and cook for 20 minutes, stirring often, until caramelized
and dark golden brown. This step is very important, as the color of the
onions at this stage will determine the color of the final product. Stir in
the garlic and flour and cook, stirring constantly, for 1–2 minutes.

Add the white wine and stir the mixture until the flour has blended in smoothly. Bring to a boil slowly, stirring constantly. Whisk or briskly stir in the stock or water. Add the bouquet garni and season with salt and freshly ground black pepper, then remove the bouquet garni. Simmer gently for 30 minutes and then remove the bouquet garni. Skim the surface of excess fat, if necessary. Add the sherry to the soup and adjust the seasoning to taste.

To make the croûtes, toast the bread slices under the broiler until dry and golden on both sides.

Ladle the soup into warm, broiler-proof bowls and float the croûtes on the top of each one. Sprinkle with the grated Gruyère and place under a preheated broiler until the cheese melts and becomes golden brown. Serve immediately.

*A bouquet garni is an aromatic blend of herbs bundled in cheesecloth and used to flavor stock. Parsley, thyme, and bay leaf would be perfect for this recipe.

NUTRITIONAL ANALYSIS PER SERVING	Calories	345	Fiber	3 g
	Carbohydrates	32 g	Protein	16 g
	Sugar	7 g	Calcium	337 mg
	Total Fat	14.6 g	Vitamin A	990 I.U.
	Saturated Fat	8 g	Vitamin C	20 mg
	Cholesterol	40 mg	Folate	57 mcg
	Sodium	371 mg		

AVEC PANACHE'S PHILOSOPHY AND DINING TIPS

Avec Panache believes in eating a balanced diet and including exercise in your lifestyle. Butter, salt, and cream are not necessarily unhealthy when used in moderation.

THE THRILL OF THE GRILL

Surfside Skewers

Serves: 4

20 Nantucket sea scallops
1 cup cubed red pepper
½ cup cubed onion
1 cup sliced mushroom or summer
   squash
¼ cup light teriyaki marinade
⅛ teaspoon ground ginger
4 large skewers

Place teriyaki marinade and ginger in a small bowl and mix well. Place scallops and vegetable pieces on skewers until you have 5 scallops and choice of vegetables on the skewer. Place skewers in a deep pan and drizzle the teriyaki sauce over each one. Let stand in refrigerator for 10 minutes or more. Place on grill for 10–15 minutes or until tender and cooked through.

NUTRITIONAL ANALYSIS PER SERVING				
	Calories	103	Fiber	1 g
	Carbohydrates	10 g	Protein	15 g
	Sugar	4 g	Calcium	26 mg
	Total Fat	0.8 g	Vitamin A	1,204 I.U.
	Saturated Fat	0.1 g	Vitamin C	75 mg
	Cholesterol	25 mg	Folate	25 mcg
	Sodium	443 mg		

Fishermen's Feast

B

Serves: 4

12 ounces sole filets
6 ounces shrimp, peeled and deveined
1 cup tomato cut in wedges
½ cup chopped red onion
⅓ cup fat-free creamy Italian dressing
   or favorite fat-free dressing
Dash of fresh pepper or favorite
   seasoning
Nonstick cooking spray

Place sole filets and shrimp with tomato and chopped onion on large sheet of heavy-duty aluminum foil sprayed with nonstick cooking spray. Cradle sides of foil around fish, shrimp, and vegetables and cover with fat-free creamy Italian dressing. Sprinkle with seasoning. Close top of aluminum foil over fish. Refrigerate for 15 minutes or more. Place on grill. Grill in foil for 15 minutes or until fish is flaky and shrimp is pink. This dish can also be prepared in the oven; bake at 375 degrees for 15–20 minutes.

NUTRITIONAL ANALYSIS PER SERVING				
Calories	172	Fiber	1 g
Carbohydrates	12 g	Protein	25 g
Sugar	5 g	Calcium	46 mg
Total Fat	1.9 g	Vitamin A	480 I.U.
Saturated Fat	0.4 g	Vitamin C	9 mg
Cholesterol	105 mg	Folate	19 mcg
Sodium	355 mg		

Off-Island Gourmet

CANDLE 79, NEW YORK CITY

The Candle 79 motto has always been "Food from farm to table." The establishment is an extension of restaurateurs Joy Pierson and Bart Potenza's dedication to a healthier world.

Joy Pierson has written and lectured extensively about food and nutrition. A magna cum laude graduate of Tufts University with twenty years of experience as a nutritional counselor, she regularly leads workshops including, most recently, a series at Whole Foods. As a spokesperson on vegetarian eating, she has appeared on Good Day New York, CBS News This Morning, *and the* Food Network's *TV Food Diners.*

Bart Potenza has written and lectured on diet and health since the mid-1970s. He has become a major spokesperson for the health food industry. Together at Candle 79 Joy and Bart infuse the Upper East Side dining scene with healthful, palate-pleasing vegetarian cuisine consisting of a seasonal array of organic ingredients.

Apple-Butternut Squash Soup

Serves: 8

⅛ cup grapeseed oil
½ cup chopped yellow onion
2 guajillo chilies
1 clove
1 cinnamon stick or 1 teaspoon
    ground cinnamon
2 bay leaves
4 cups peeled and chopped butternut
    squash (approx. 1 squash)
1 16-ounce bottle Nantucket Nectars®
    Cloudy Apple juice
3 quarts water or vegetable stock
¼ cup maple syrup
2 tablespoons fresh sage
Salt to taste

Over medium-high heat, heat oil, add onion and spices, and sauté 2–3 minutes. Add squash and apple juice; simmer for 5 minutes. Add water or stock and bring to a boil; reduce to simmer and cook until squash is tender (approximately 30 minutes). Remove from heat and add maple syrup, fresh sage, and salt to taste. Blend in blender until very smooth, and serve.

NUTRITIONAL ANALYSIS PER SERVING	Calories	133	Fiber	3 g
	Carbohydrates	26 g	Protein	1 g
	Sugar	15 g	Calcium	62 mg
	Total Fat	3.6 g	Vitamin A	12,045 I.U.
	Saturated Fat	0.4 g	Vitamin C	17 mg
	Cholesterol	0 mg	Folate	22 mcg
	Sodium	7 mg		

Tofu Spring Rolls

Serves: 8

½ pound extra-firm tofu, cut into 6
    pieces
1 cup wheat vermicelli, cooked
Juice from 1 lime
2 tablespoons minced ginger
⅛ cup tamari
⅛ cup brown rice vinegar
1 tablespoon chili paste or hot sauce
    of choice
1½ teaspoons organic sugar
2 scallions, sliced
1½ teaspoons sesame oil
½ cucumber
½ mango
½ tablespoon cilantro

½ tablespoon basil
½ tablespoon mint
8 small pieces rice paper
2 tablespoons Avocado Dipping Sauce
(recipe follows)

Mix together lime juice, ginger, tamari, vinegar, chili paste, sugar, scallions, and oil. This is the marinade. Lay tofu slices in baking dish and cover with marinade. Bake uncovered at 350 degrees for 30 minutes. Soak rice paper in bowl of hot water until edges soften. Remove from bowl. Shake off any excess water, place on flat surface, and blot dry.

Slice tofu into desired size. Combine with vermicelli, thinly sliced cucumbers, scallions, mango; cilantro, basil, and mint; roll in rice paper. To serve, cut spring rolls into 2 pieces and serve with Avocado Dipping Sauce.

NUTRITIONAL ANALYSIS PER SERVING	Calories	110	Fiber	3 g
	Carbohydrates	13 g	Protein	5 g
	Sugar	0 g	Calcium	35 mg
	Total Fat	5.6 g	Vitamin A	105 I.U.
	Saturated Fat	0.8 g	Vitamin C	2 mg
	Cholesterol	0 mg	Folate	18 mcg
	Sodium	382 mg		

Avocado Dipping Sauce

A

Serves: 8

1 avocado, sliced
½ cup water
Juice and zest from 1 lime
¼ cup Nantucket Nectars® Orange-
Cranberry juice
1 teaspoon minced ginger

1 jalapeño pepper, chopped
1 teaspoon salt

Blend all ingredients together in blender until smooth.

NUTRITIONAL ANALYSIS PER SERVING				
Calories	47	Fiber	2 g
Carbohydrates	4 g	Protein	1 g
Sugar	2 g	Calcium	4 mg
Total Fat	3.7 g	Vitamin A	53 I.U.
Saturated Fat	0.5 g	Vitamin C	7 mg
Cholesterol	0 mg	Folate	16 mcg
Sodium	297 mg		

Chocolate Cake with Raspberry Sauce

A "Make Love to Life" Dessert

 Serves: 12

1 cup unbleached white flour
1 cup pastry flour
2 teaspoons baking powder
2 teaspoons baking soda
½ cup cocoa powder
1 teaspoon salt
½ teaspoon cinnamon
½ cup Sucanat®
½ cup water
1 cup soy milk
1 cup maple syrup
½ cup safflower oil
2 teaspoons apple cider vinegar
1 teaspoon vanilla extract
½ teaspoon almond extract

½ bottle Nantucket Nectars®
  raspberry juice
1 cup Nantucket Nectars® apple juice
½ cup organic sugar
2 cups frozen or fresh raspberries

Preheat the oven to 350 degrees. Mix the flours, baking powder, baking soda, cocoa powder, salt, cinnamon, and Sucanat® together in a large mixing bowl. Mix the water, soy milk, maple syrup, oil, vinegar, and vanilla and almond extracts together in another bowl. Pour the wet ingredients into the flour mixture and stir well to combine. Divide the batter into 2 greased 9-inch cake pans. Bake for 35 minutes or until a cake tester or toothpick comes out clean. Remove from oven and let cool on wire racks for about 30 minutes.

Over medium-high heat, cook raspberry juice, apple juice, and sugar until reduced by half. Add raspberries and remove from heat. Transfer to a blender and puree until very smooth (puree can be poured through strainer if a smoother consistency is desired). To serve, ladle sauce over cake.

NUTRITIONAL ANALYSIS PER SERVING				
Calories	332	Fiber	3 g
Carbohydrates	58 g	Protein	4 g
Sugar	35 g	Calcium	86 mg
Total Fat	10.3 g	Vitamin A	21 I.U.
Saturated Fat	0.9 g	Vitamin C	8 mg
Cholesterol	0 mg	Folate	19 mcg
Sodium	303 mg		

JASPER WHITE'S SUMMER SHACK, BOSTON

World-renowned chef Jasper White's Summer Shack, specializes in contemporary and traditional New England fare and seafood. The flavors of the food and the variety of classic dishes reflect the true simplicity and rustic feel of the restaurant, designed to look like a coastal clam shack. The Summer Shack brings a refreshing, fun dining atmosphere to neighbors and visitors of Boston alike.

The philosophy behind Jasper White's Summer Shack is "Food is love," and the proof is in the dishes. Jasper White is the author of highly praised cookbooks. He has won numerous awards, including the James Beard Award for Best Chef in the Northeast and Food and Wine's Honor Roll of American Chefs.

Broiled Nantucket Cape Scallops with Garlic, Parsley, and Butter

Late fall is peak season for Nantucket cape scallops—the sweetest scallops on the planet. The recipe is simple, allowing for the true flavor of the scallops to dominate.

Serves: 4

1½ pounds fresh cape scallops
1 tablespoon olive oil
2 teaspoons minced fresh garlic
1 teaspoon kosher or sea salt
¼ teaspoon freshly ground black
    pepper
¼ cup white wine
¼ cup chopped parsley
4 tablespoons unsalted butter, softened

Pick through the scallops, and remove the straps and any bits of shell. Distribute the scallops on several layers of paper towels and dry well.

Adjust the oven rack to the broiler position and preheat the broiler. Place a large platter in the oven to warm. While the broiler is heating, transfer the dry scallops to a medium bowl and toss them well with the olive oil, garlic, salt, and pepper (clean fingers work best). Remove the platter and place a sheet pan under the broiler, allowing it to get very hot.

Quickly place the scallops in a single layer on the sheet pan so most of them are not touching. You will hear them sizzle. Broil 3½ inches from the source of heat without turning until the scallops are opaque, about 2 minutes. Remove the sheet pan from the broiler and drizzle the scallops with white wine to loosen the drippings from the pan. Quickly place them in a bowl with the softened butter and parsley. Toss them with a spatula so they are well coated with the garlic, parsley, and butter.

Transfer the scallops to the warm platter, and serve immediately over cooked whole-wheat pasta or brown rice, 1 cup (not included in analysis) adds 175 calories for pasta and 215 for rice (optional).

NUTRITIONAL ANALYSIS PER SERVING				
	Calories	294	Fiber	0 g
	Carbohydrates	5 g	Protein	29 g
	Sugar	0 g	Calcium	51 mg
	Total Fat	15.7 g	Vitamin A	802 I.U.
	Saturated Fat	7.6 g	Vitamin C	11 mg
	Cholesterol	86 mg	Folate	33 mcg
	Sodium	748 mg		

ESTIMATING PORTION SIZE

FOOD	OBJECT
1 serving of vegetables or fruit	Your fist
An apple	A baseball
A potato	A computer mouse
3 ounces of meat, fish, or poultry	A deck of cards, or your palm (without fingers)
1 cup cooked pasta or rice	Your fist
1 ounce of cheese	4 stacked dice or your whole thumb
½ cup ice cream	A tennis ball
A bagel	A hockey puck
*A pancake	A compact disc
A muffin	A racquetball
1 ounce nuts or small candy	The palm of your hand
1 serving of cereal	A tennis ball
1 serving of snacks such as pretzel, chips, etc.	A cupped handful
2 tablespoons margarine, peanut butter, cream cheese, etc.	A thumb, joint to tip
1 teaspoon of oil, extract, etc.	The tip of your thumb

To gain perspective on how much food is in a recommended serving size, the following information from the USDA may prove to be helpful.[1]

1 SERVING EQUALS:

- 1 slice of whole-grain bread
- ½ cup of cooked rice or pasta
- ½ cup of mashed potatoes
- ½ cup of cooked or raw vegetables
- 1 small baked potato
- 1 cup of lettuce
- 1 medium apple
- ½ cup of berries
- ½ grapefruit or mango
- ¾ cup of vegetable juice
- 1½ ounces of cheddar cheese
- 1 cup of yogurt or milk
- 1 chicken breast (3–4 ounces)
- 1 medium pork chop
- ¼ pound hamburger patty
- 1 small pancake or waffle
- 3–4 small crackers
- 2 medium-sized cookies

CALORIE COUNTER

	Calories
Alcohol	
Beer, 12 ounces	145
Beer, light, 12 ounces	95
Champagne, 3 ounces	75
Gin, rum, vodka, whiskey, 1.5 ounces, 80 proof	95
Gin, rum, vodka, whiskey, 1.5 ounces, 90 proof	110
Liqueurs, 1 ounce	90
Wine, dessert, 3.5 ounces	140
Wine, red, 3.5 ounces	70
Wine, white, 3.5 ounces	80
Beverages	
Coffee, 6 ounces	0
Coffee, iced, without sugar, 6 ounces	0
Coffee, instant, flavored, 6 ounces	5
Hot chocolate, diet, 1 packet	25
Hot chocolate, regular, 1 packet	80
Hot chocolate, sugar-free, 1 packet	40
Tea, 6 ounces	0
Tea, iced, without sugar, 6 ounces	0
Bread	
Bagel, 1 average	200
Bread crumbs, 1 cup	390
Bread sticks, 4 pieces	50
Bread stuffing mix, 2 cups	250
Bun, hamburger or hot dog	115
Croissant, 1 medium	180
Croutons, 2 tablespoons	30
Dinner roll	130
Doughnuts, 1 plain cake	210
Doughnuts, 1 raised glazed	235
English muffin	130
French bread, 1 slice	80

	Calories
Italian bread, 1 slice	60
Light bread, all varieties, 1 slice	40
Muffin, 1 average	180
Muffin, 1 average light or small	90
Multigrain bread, 1 slice	70
Oatmeal bread, 1 slice	65
Pancakes, frozen, light, 3 pancakes	190
Pita pocket, 53 g	140
Pita pocket, mini, 28 g	80
Pizza, 1 slice	290
Pumpernickel bread, 1 slice	80
Raisin bread, 1 slice	70
Taco shell, 1	70
Tortilla, flour, 43 g	130
Waffle, fat-free, 2	160
Waffle, frozen, 2	190
White bread, 1 slice	60
Cereal	
All-Bran with Extra Fiber, ½ cup	50
Bran flakes, ¾ cup	90
Cocoa Krispies, ¾ cup	120
Cocoa Puffs, 1 cup	120
Corn Pops, 1 cup	110
Cornflakes, 1 cup	100
Cream of Wheat, 3 tablespoons	120
Granola, low-fat with raisins, ⅔ cup	210
Multigrain Flakes, 1 cup	100
Oatmeal, ½ cup dry	150
Puffed rice, 1 cup	60
Puffed wheat, 1 cup	50
Raisin bran, 1 cup	170
Toasted oat cereal, 1 cup	110
Condiments and Pickles	
Bread and butter pickles, 4 slices	20

CALORIE COUNTER

Dill chips, 5	5	Cream cheese, 2 tablespoons	100
Ketchup, 1 tablespoon	15	Cream cheese, fat-free,	
Mayonnaise, 1 tablespoon	100	2 tablespoons	30
Mayonnaise, light, 1 tablespoon	50	Cream cheese, light,	
Mustard, 1 teaspoon	5	2 tablespoons	60
Mustard (honey mustard),		Feta, ¼ cup	95
1 teaspoon	10	Gruyère, 1 ounce	115
Sweet gherkins, small, 1	20	Mozzarella, fat-free, ¼ cup	45
Sweet pickle chips, 5 chips	40	Mozzarella, part-skim, 1 ounce	80
Cooking Ingredients		Muenster, 1 ounce	105
Baking powder, 1 teaspoon	3	Neufchâtel, 1 ounce	75
Cocoa powder, tablespoon	14	Parmesan, 1 tablespoon	25
Cornstarch, 1 tablespoon	30	Provolone, 1 ounce	100
Cream of Tartar, 1 teaspoon	2	Ricotta, fat-free, ½ cup	120
Flavor extracts:		Ricotta, reduced-fat, ½ cup	200
- Imitation, 1 teaspoon	5	Romano, 1 tablespoon	25
- Pure almond or vanilla,		Swiss, 1 ounce	105
1 teaspoon	10	Swiss, light, low-salt, 1 ounce	90
- All other varieties, 1 teaspoon	20	CREAM:	
Vinegar, 1 ounce	4	Half-and-half, 1 tablespoon	20
Yeast, dry, ¼ ounce	20	Heavy, 1 tablespoon	50
Dairy Products		Imitation dry creamers, 1 teaspoon	10
Butter, 1 tablespoon	100	Imitation liquid mini creamer,	
Margarine, 1 tablespoon	45	1 container	15
Margarine, spray, 5 sprays	5	Imitation whipped cream,	
Margarine, squeezable, non-fat,		1 tablespoon	10
1 tablespoon	5	Sour cream, 1 tablespoon	30
CHEESE:		Light, 1 tablespoon	30
American, 1 ounce	105	Light sour cream, 1 tablespoon	20
American, fat-free, 1 slice	30	ICE CREAM:	
Blue, 1 ounce	100	Creamsicle, sugar-free	30
Camembert, 1 wedge	115	Frozen yogurt, ½ cup	100
Cheddar, 1 ounce	115	Fudgesicle, sugar-free	45
Cheddar, fat-free, 1 slice	35	Ice-cream cone, sugar, 1	40
Cottage, 2%, 1 cup	200	Ice-cream cone, waffle cup, 1	20
Cottage, low-fat, 1 cup	80	Ice-cream sandwich, fat-free	130

CALORIE COUNTER

Light, fat-free, ½ cup	100	Lobster, raw, 3 ounces	75
Sherbet, ½ cup	130	Mussels, cooked, 3 ounces	75
Soft-serve, ½ cup	110	Oysters, raw, ½ cup (6 to 10	
Sorbet, ½ cup	110	medium)	80
10% fat, all flavors, ½ cup	140	Roe, 3 ounces	120
MILK:		Salmon, baked or smoked,	
Buttermilk, 1 cup	100	3 ounces	140
Evaporated, skim, 1 cup	200	Scallops, 3 ounces	75
Low-fat milk (2%), 1 cup	120	Scallops, raw, 2 large or 5 small	25
Skim milk, 1 cup	90	Shrimp, 3 ounces	90
Soy milk, 1 cup	70	Shrimp, cooked, 4 large	30
Whole milk, 1 cup	150	Snapper, cooked, 4 ounces	115

Dip

		Sole, cooked, 3 ounces	80
Dip, light, fat-free, 2 tablespoons	30	Squid, 4 ounces	105
Dip, most varieties, 2 tablespoons	60	Striped bass, raw, 1 fillet	125
Guacamole, 2 tablespoons	50	Swordfish, raw, 3 ounces	130
Hummus, 2 tablespoons	50	Tuna, packed in water, 1 can,	
Pâté, 2 tablespoons	60	6 ounces	220
Salsa, 2 tablespoons	20	Tuna, packed in water, 3 ounces	108
Tahini, 2 tablespoons	180	Tuna, raw, 4 ounces	140

Dressings, Salad

Flour

Light, 2 tablespoons	30	Soy, 1 cup	400
Most varieties, 2 tablespoons	100	Wheat, 1 cup	400
Sugar-free, fat-free, 2 tablespoons	0	White all-purpose, 1 cup	440

Fish and Shellfish

Fruit

Bluefish, raw, 1 fillet	155	Apple, 1 medium	80
Caviar (black or red), 1 tablespoon	40	Applesauce, sweetened, 4 ounces	95
Clams, raw, 3 ounces	65	Applesauce, unsweetened,	
Crab, Alaskan king, raw, 4 ounces	95	4 ounces	50
Crab, blue, raw, 3 ounces	75	Apricot, 1	20
Fish stock, 1 cup	40	Avocado, peeled, 1	170
Flounder, raw, 3 ounces	80	Banana, 1 medium	105
Haddock, raw, 3 ounces	100	Blackberries, 1 cup	60
Halibut, raw, 3 ounces	110	Blueberries, 1 cup	80
Lobster, edible portion of one whole,		Cantaloupe, ½ of 5-inch-diameter	
1 pound	135	melon	45

CALORIE COUNTER

Cherries, 1 cup	90	**Dried Fruits**	
Coconut, dried, sweetened, ½ cup	185	Apricots, 5	100
Coconut, flesh, 1 ounce	100	Cranberries, ⅓ cup	130
Cranberries, 1 cup	60	Dates, 10 (½ cup)	240
Grapefruit, ½ medium	40	Figs, 10	475
Grapes, 1 cup	90	Prunes, 5 large	115
Honeydew melon, 1 cup	60	Raisins, 1 cup	435
Kiwi, 1	45	Raisins, 1 mini box, 14 g	45
Lemon, 1	15	**Herbs, Spices, Seasonings**	
Lime, 1	20	Allspice, 1 teaspoon	5
Mango, 1	135	Bacon bits, 1 tablespoon	30
Nectarine, 1	65	Basil, fresh, 2 tablespoons	1
Orange, 1	60	Bouillon cubes, 1 cube	15
Peach, 1	35	Butter Buds, 1 teaspoon	5
Pear, Bartlett, 1	100	Cheese sprinkles, imitation,	
Pear, Bosc, 1	85	1 teaspoon	5
Pear, D'Anjou, 1	120	Chili powder, 1 teaspoon	8
Pineapple, 1 cup	75	Chives, fresh, 2 tablespoons	1
Plum, 1	35	Cinnamon, 1 teaspoon	6
Raspberries, 1 cup	60	Cloves, 1 teaspoon	6
Strawberries, 1 cup	50	Curry powder, 1 teaspoon	6
Tangerines, 1	35	Garlic, raw, 1 clove	4
Watermelon, 1 cup	40	Ginger, 1 teaspoon	6
Fruit Juices (per 8-ounce serving)		Nutmeg, 1 teaspoon	12
Cranberry	145	Onion powder, 1 teaspoon	7
Cranberry, light	40	Oregano, 1 teaspoon	5
Grape	155	Paprika, 1 teaspoon	5
Grapefruit	95	Parsley, dried, 1 teaspoon	4
Grapefruit, light	40	Parsley, fresh, 10 sprigs	5
Lemon	60	Pepper (black, red, white),	
Lime	65	1 teaspoon	6
Orange	110	Peppermint, fresh, 2 tablespoons	2
Orange, light	50	Rosemary, 1 teaspoon	5
Pineapple	140	Saffron, 1 teaspoon	2
Prune	180	Salt, 1 teaspoon	0
Tomato	40	Thyme, dried, 1 teaspoon	3

CALORIE COUNTER

Turmeric, 1 teaspoon	8	Pecans, ½ cup	360

Honey, Jams, and Preserves

Honey, 1 tablespoon	65
Jam and preserves, 1 tablespoon	55
Jam and preserves, sugar-free, 1 tablespoon	10
Jellies, 1 tablespoon	50
Jellies, sugar-free, 1 tablespoon	10

Meat

Bacon:	
Canadian style, 2 slices	85
Crisp strips, low-salt, 3 slices	110
Beef cuts, cooked:	
Flank steak, 3 ounces	220
Ground beef, lean, 3 ounces	235
Pot roast, 3 ounces	195
Rib roast, 3 ounces	205
Sirloin steak, lean, 3 ounces	200
Bologna, 2 slices	180
Frankfurter, 1	150
Ham, 3 ounce	195
Ham, deli slices, 2	60
Lamb, 3 ounces	245
Pork chop, lean, 3 ounces	200
Salami, 2 slices	85
Sausage, 2 links	130
Veal, 3 ounces	190

Nuts

Almonds, 1 ounce	165
Brazil nuts, 1 ounce	185
Cashews, 1 ounce	165
Hazelnuts, ½ cup	360
Macadamia, ½ cup	480
Mixed nuts, 1 ounce	170
Peanuts, ¼ cup	165
Peanut butter, 1 tablespoon	95
Pecans, ½ cup	360
Pine nuts, 1 ounce	160
Pistachio, 1 ounce	165
Soy nuts, 1 ounce	150
Walnuts, 1 ounce	170

Oil

Corn, 1 tablespoon	120
Grapeseed, 1 tablespoon	125
Olive, 1 tablespoon	120
Peanut, 1 tablespoon	125
Soybean, 1 tablespoon	125
Sunflower, 1 tablespoon	120
Vegetable, 1 tablespoon	120
Walnut, 1 tablespoon	125

Pasta

Angel hair, fresh, cooked, 1¼ cups	240
Elbows, 2 ounces	220
Elbows, cooked, 1 cup	155
Fettuccine, fresh, cooked, 1¼ cups	250
Lasagna, dry, 2 ounces	210
Linguine, dry, 2 ounces	210
Noodles, fresh, cooked, 1 cup	220
Ravioli, cheese, frozen, 6 large	360
Spaghetti, dry, 2 ounces	210
Tortellini, 1 cup	230
Whole-wheat, cooked, 1 cup	175

Poultry

Chicken, 3 ounces:	
Breast, skinless, baked	120
Drumstick, skinless, baked	130
Thigh, skinless, baked	150
Wing, skinless, baked	150
Chicken, deli slices, 1 slice	20
Chicken dog (frankfurter)	50
Chicken noodle soup, canned, 1 cup	75

CALORIE COUNTER

Turkey, 3 ounces:	
Breast, skinless, baked	120
Drumstick, skinless, baked	140
Thigh, skinless, baked	140
Turkey bacon, 1 slice	35
Turkey ground, 4 ounces	112
Turkey sausage, 1 link	70
Turkey slices, 2 slices	40
Pudding	
Prepared, ½ cup	140
Prepared from:	
Sugar-free mix, ½ cup	70
Snack size, 4 ounces	80
Rice	
Brown, long grain, cooked, 1 cup	215
Brown, long grain, uncooked,	
¼ cup	150
Risotto, 1 cup	420
White, instant, cooked, 1 cup	180
White, uncooked, ¼ cup	150
Wild, uncooked, ½ cup	110
Sauce	
A-1, 1 tablespoon	15
Alfredo, ¼ cup	290
Cranberry, ½ cup	160
Marinara, ½ cup	80
Pesto, ¼ cup	140
Seafood cocktail sauce, ¼ cup	100
Soy, 1 tablespoon	10
Spaghetti, light, ½ cup	50
Spaghetti, most varieties,	
½ cup	100
Tabasco, 1 teaspoon	5
Tartar sauce, 2 tablespoons	80
Tartar sauce, low fat,	
2 tablespoons	40

Teriyaki, marinade, 1 tablespoon	25
Worcestershire, 1 tablespoon	10
Seeds	
Anise, 1 teaspoon	7
Fenugreek, 1 teaspoon	12
Mustard, 1 teaspoon	15
Other, 1 teaspoon	7
Poppy, 1 teaspoon	15
Pumpkin, ¼ cup	70
Sesame, 1 teaspoon	16
Sunflower, ¼ cup	80
Snacks	
Cheese Nips® crackers,	
29 crackers	150
Cracker Jack®, 1 box	120
Graham crackers, 1 sheet	60
Melba toast, 3 slices	60
Popcorn, air-popped, no salt,	
1 cup	20
Potato chips, 10 chips	105
Potato chips, fat-free, 15 chips	70
Pretzels, 10 sticks	10
Rice cakes, 1 average cake	60
Ritz® crackers, 5 crackers	80
Saltines, 5 crackers	60
Soy crisps, 25 crisps	100
Soy tortilla chips, 15 chips	140
Tortilla chips, 18 chips	140
Triscuits™, 7 crackers	140
Veggie chips, 21 chips	140
Wasa® crispbread (crackers),	
1 piece	30
Wheat Thins™, 4 crackers	70
Soy	
Soy bacon, 2 slices	45
Soy dog (frankfurter), 1	60

CALORIE COUNTER

Sugar

Brown, 1 teaspoon	15
Powdered, sifted, 1 cup	385
White, 1 teaspoon	15
White, ¼ cup	180

Sweets

Boxed chocolates, 1 piece	80
Brownie, 1 average (61 gram)	270
Caramels, 1 piece	40
Chocolate chip cookie, 1 average (15 grams)	80
Chocolate-covered peanuts, 16 pieces	210
Chocolate-covered raisins, 34 pieces	170
Fig Newton cookies, 2 cookies	110
Fudge, 1 ounce	115
Fudge with nuts, 1 ounce	120
Gelatin, all flavors, ½ cup	80
Gelatin, sugar-free, ½ cup	10
Halvah, 1 ounce	160
Hard candy, 1 piece	20
Hershey® Kisses, 1 piece	25
Jelly beans, 10 small	100
Licorice, 1 piece	25
Marshmallow Fluff, 1 ounce	90
Marshmallows, 2 pieces	90
Meringue cookies, 4 cookies	90
M&M's, 1 peanut	10
M&M's, 1 plain	4
Oatmeal raisin cookie, 1 average (15 g)	70
Peanut brittle, 1 ounce	130
Peanut butter cup, 1 piece	100
Pecan Sandies, 1 cookie	80

Syrup

Chocolate, 2 tablespoons	100
Chocolate, light, 2 tablespoons	50
Chocolate, sugar-free, 2 tablespoons	15
Corn, 2 tablespoons	170
Grenadine, 2 tablespoons	55
Karo™, ½ cup	240
Maple:	
- Calorie-reduced, ¼ cup	60
- Pure, ¼ cup	210
- Sugar-free ¼ cup	2
Molasses, 2 tablespoons	85

Tofu

Tofu, ⅕ of package (79 g)	85
Tofu, light, ⅕ of package (79 g)	40

Vegetables

Alfalfa sprouts, ½ cup	5
Artichokes, ½ cup	40
Asparagus, 4 spears	15
Bean sprouts, 1 cup	30
Beans:	
Black, 1 cup	225
Butter, ½ cup	90
Green, 1 cup	40
Kidney, red, canned, ½ cup	115
Lima, cooked, 1 cup	260
Navy, dry, cooked, 1 cup	117
Pinto, cooked, 1 cup	225
Soybean, cooked, ½ cup	105
Yellow wax, 1 cup	40
Beets, cooked, 1 cup	50
Black-eyed peas, 1 cup	190
Broccoli, 1 cup	50
Brussels sprouts, 1 cup	60

CALORIE COUNTER

Cabbage:		Onions, red, 1 cup	20
Chinese, 1 cup	20	Parsnips, 1 cup	125
Common, 1 cup	15	Peas, cooked, ¼ cup	35
Carrots, 1 cup	70	Peas, raw with pods,	
Cauliflower, 1 cup	30	½ pound	70
Celery, 1 cup	20	Peppers:	
Celery, 1 stalk	5	Green, raw, 1 cup	20
Chickpeas, 1 cup	270	Hot chili, 1	20
Corn:		Red, raw, 1 cup	20
1 ear, cooked	85	Potatoes:	
½ cup cooked	85	Baked with skin, 1	220
½ cup creamed	95	Boiled, flesh only, 1	120
Cucumber, ½ medium	15	French fries, 10	150
Cucumbers, 6 slices	5	Radishes, 4	5
Eggplant, steamed, 1 cup	25	Seaweed, dried, 1 ounce	50
Kale, 1 cup	40	Snow peas (8–9 pods)	10
Lentils, 1 cup	215	Spinach, 1 cup	10
Lettuce:		Squash, summer, cooked, 1 cup	35
Crisp head, 1 cup	5	Squash, winter, ½ cup	40
Crisp head, 1 head	70	Sweet potato, baked, peeled, 1	115
Loose-leaf, 1 cup	10	Sweet potato, candied, mashed,	
Mushrooms, 1 cup	20	1 cup	260
Nori, leaves, dried, 6 sheets	35	Tomatoes, 1 average	25
Olives, black, 1 large	15	Turnip, diced, cooked, 1 cup	30
Olives, green, 3 small	15	Yams, cooked, ½ cup	80
Onions, 1 cup sliced	40	Zucchini, ½ cup	13

Chapter 10

JANE'S EXERCISE TIPS FOR A LIFETIME OF FITNESS AND CARDIOVASCULAR HEALTH

*E*xercise plays a key role in weight loss and weight mainte-nance. It not only makes a diet plan more successful, it aids in producing several important health benefits, including reducing the risk of heart disease and high blood pressure, lowering cholesterol, and reducing insulin resistance. Regular exercise may reduce the risk of many common cancers. It helps to decrease stress, ward off anxiety and depression, promote healthy sleep patterns, and even reduce some of the effects of aging. Making exercise a part of your life improves circulation and flexibility and increases energy and endurance levels. Exer-cise also helps build and maintain muscle mass, which is an especially significant factor for those at risk of osteoporosis. Engaging in a consistent exercise program allows you to main-tain an appropriate body weight. Successes gained through exer-cise also contribute to increased confidence and self-esteem. The benefits of exercise are so significant that if it is not already a part of your daily life, it should be.

Cardiovascular disease is the number one killer in America, accounting for hundreds of thousands of deaths per year, many of which may be attributable to lack of regular exercise.[1] The American Heart Association has added lack of exercise to its list of major risk factors for heart disease. A sedentary lifestyle is as dangerous as smoking a pack of cigarettes a day. Heart disease is almost twice as likely to develop in inactive people. Regular exercise is vital to good cardiovascular health. It is a key component in the prevention and treatment of heart disease.

Participation in regular physical activity gradually increased during the 1960s, 1970s, and 1980s but seems to have leveled off in recent years.[2] Surveys show that almost one-third of Americans eighteen or older are not active at all. Most people recognize the value of physical activity and exercise for the human body, yet it is estimated that 40 percent of the American population is completely inactive.[3] Almost half of all adults report some exercise but do not exercise regularly or intensely enough to derive any cardiac benefit. Less than one-third of Americans get enough exercise to achieve cardiovascular fitness. Another significant fact is that the dropout rate for those who do start an exercise program reaches 50 percent or more by the conclusion of the first six months.[4]

Motivation and self-control are essential elements in weight management and exercise. Motivation is required to get you started and committed to making changes in your lifestyle. As you begin to see results, no matter how small they are, continuing toward your goal becomes increasingly less difficult. On a personal note, I am one of those individuals who does not always enjoy exercising; drive and dedication are the only forces that have helped me to reach my goals.

There are some key motivating techniques that will make your decision to begin a workout program and to remain on it a bit easier.

- **Visualization.** Imagine yourself at 10, 20, 30 pounds lighter. Actually picture yourself at a lower weight in your mind, and use this as an incentive to work toward your goal.

- **Realism.** Set attainable goals. Do not believe that you can lose weight and get in shape in just a week. It may take at least a month to see any noticeable changes. You may also find a level at which you plateau. You need not get discouraged; making changes in your exercise routine will help you surpass it.

- **Health.** Exercise and weight loss can have incredible long-term health benefits. This can be enough of a motivating factor for many people.

- **Target date.** Choose a particular event you may be attending—a reunion or a wedding, for example—that you wish to lose weight for and use it as a goal date.

- **Role models and group support.** Ask someone who has been successful at getting and staying in shape for advice. Look to friends and family for positive reinforcement.

- **Plotting success.** Keep a journal to see the positive results of your hard work.

- **Just rewards.** With each success gained, make sure to reward yourself with something special.

Discipline is essential when trying to follow your exercise program consistently. In order to remain on an exercise regimen, it needs to be not only effective but enjoyable. Many people lose interest because their workout choices become boring. The way to counteract this problem is to change your routine. If bike riding feels like it's becoming a chore, for instance, change to walking or jogging. Music is a great motivator. Incorporating indoor as well as outdoor activities keeps things interesting. Setting new goals can also be helpful. Instead of planning to work out for a certain amount of time, target a particular number of calories that you want to burn or number of miles that you want to cover on that day.

For those of you who really hate working out, there are some activities that you can engage in that won't even seem like exercise. Spend a night out dancing. Just make sure that most of your time is spent on the dance floor and not at the bar (unless you are getting water). It is possible to burn 572 calories in two hours without even realizing it. Many people off-island walk the local malls to exercise. On the island, take advantage of the harbor docks. Walking up and down viewing the magnificent yachts will help keep you moving without even a thought of exercise. Window-shopping serves the same purpose; you can walk along the cobblestone streets looking in the windows of all the wonderful boutiques, art galleries, and antiques stores. Walking Nantucket's endless stretch of beaches is also a perfect way to burn some calories. You will be amazed at how many miles of beach you can cover without even being aware of it.

You will see from the exercise chart on page 267 that fishing is a great activity that even burns calories. An added benefit is that you can bring home the main ingredient for a wonderful low-calorie dinner. For individuals who are tired of traffic, get on your bike—you may arrive at your destination faster than you would if you were driving. The point here is that even if you think you're an exercise-hater, feeling like you have a purpose to your activity may make it a lot easier to bear. As you can see, no matter where you live, there are options that will keep you moving.

Knowing and appreciating your workout personality will make it easier for you to remain committed. Typically, individuals fall into four categories. Type I includes those who like the gym setting. Type IIs are people who wish to create an at-home gym and work out privately. Type III individuals are competitors and thus like to engage in team sports such as volleyball, racquetball, and soccer. Type IV is the socialite who enjoys walking with friends or enrolling in class situations such as dance, aerobics, or yoga.

You should designate a block of time in your day that is convenient for you to exercise. Some people find that the morning is the best time for them. Others choose lunchtime or after work. Some may never have a period that is lengthy enough to complete a full workout, so they choose to split it up. They may opt to exercise twenty minutes in the morning and the same at night (but if you have difficulty sleeping, you may not want to exercise too close to your bedtime). Whatever time you choose, even if it varies, it is important to think about exercising before-hand and put it into your agenda, just like any other appointment. Thus working exercise into your daily routine becomes a habit, something that you can stick to for life.

It is essential that whatever type of exercise you choose, you include a warm-up and cool-down with stretching; this keeps your regimen safe and helps to avoid any potential injury. Remember that if you feel faint, dizzy, out of breath, or nauseated, or if you have pain, you must stop— you are overdoing it.

Before exercise, it is essential to warm up for two to five minutes, and cool down afterward for the same amount of time. This usually incorporates the exercise that you are engaging in, but at a much lower intensity; for example, if you are going to be jogging, start out by march-ing in place or walking for three minutes. This should be followed by your stretching routine.

Stretching must be conducted in a relaxed mode, without bouncing, until you feel a slight tension. The following chart illustrates ten easy stretches that can be done anywhere, anytime, in approximately five minutes.

Neck: Turn your chin toward your right shoulder. Hold the stretch for ten seconds. This stretches the left side of your neck. Then stretch the other side. Repeat twice.

Sides of upper body, shoulders, and arms: Place right arm straight up. Place left arm straight down by your side. Reach in opposite directions. Hold for twenty seconds. Repeat on the other side.

Upper back, shoulders, and arms: Raise arms straight up over your head. Lock fingers together, palms facing up; move arms slightly back and upward. Hold for twenty seconds.

Chest, shoulders, arms: Place arms in a straight position behind your back and interlock your fingers, palms up. Turn elbows inward, then lift your arms behind you until you feel a good stretch. Hold for twenty seconds.

Back: Put your hands on the back of your hips, knees slightly bent. Slowly lean back from the waist until you feel a stretch in your back. Hold for fifteen seconds. Repeat one time.

Lower back, hips, groin: Place feet straight forward and shoulder-width apart. Keeping knees slightly bent, slowly bend from waist toward the floor until you feel a stretch in the back of your legs and lower back. Hold for fifteen seconds. When finished, slowly return to an upright position.

Inner thigh: Spread legs apart with feet pointing outward. Bend left knee slightly; move right hip downward toward left knee. Hold for fifteen seconds. This stretches the right thigh. Repeat for the left thigh.

Quadriceps and knee: Hold top of your left foot with your right hand behind your back. Pull your heel toward your buttocks. Hold for twenty seconds, then repeat with the opposite foot.

Calf: Lean against a wall with your forearms, forehead resting on your hands. Bend one leg in front of you and place the other leg straight behind; keep your back flat and heels on the ground.

Move your hips forward until you feel the stretch in your calf. Hold for fifteen seconds. Repeat with the opposite leg.

Groin, ankles, Achilles tendon: Spread your feet shoulder-width apart. Place your hands inside upper legs above your knee. Lower your hips downward as you push your upper legs outward. Hold for twenty seconds.

If you have been living a sedentary lifestyle or have particular health issues, it is important that you begin at a slow pace. Your exercise routine should start at ten to twenty minutes per day, targeting a 100–250-calorie burn. A slow increase should occur to reach twenty to sixty minutes per day, burning the optimal 250–500 calories. We recommend that individuals begin exercising three times per week, working up to five times per week. Your body does need days of rest to repair muscle tissue. It has been well established that most people need to do twenty to thirty minutes of sustained exercise at least five days a week to derive full cardiovascular benefit.[5] However, every little bit of activity helps. Calories are burned not only during a scheduled workout but also doing everyday tasks such as housework, lawn care, and gardening, as well as walking to and from your car. In order to lose one pound per week, a deficit of 3,500 calories (500 calories per day) is required from either eating less, exercising more, or a combination of both. You can maximize the energy used during your daily routine by being conscious of your body in motion. The more effort that you put into the movements of your body, the more benefit your body gets out of it.

Many people choose one certain type of exercise to gain specific results. For example, practicing yoga will result in improved strength in the upper and lower body, more flexibility, better mental focus, stress reduction, and relaxation. Pilates is particularly advantageous to those desiring a more sculpted midsection as well as long, lean muscles.[6]

Even though you may have explicit fitness goals in mind, it is important to incorporate both aerobic and anaerobic activities into your routine. Aerobic exercises are those that use large muscle groups at moderate intensities; they allow the body to use oxygen to supply energy continuously for a long period.[7] Some examples of aerobic exercise include jogging, brisk walking, biking, and swimming. For the best results, you should exercise at a level strenuous enough to raise your heart rate to your target zone. To find your heart rate, place your index and middle fingers on your neck (carotid artery) or wrist and count the number of pulse beats for twenty seconds, then multiply by three to get the beats per minute.

The following formula provides a range for your target heart rate.[8] Subtract your age from 220 (the maximum heart rate), then multiply by 0.6 for the lower end (60 percent of your maximum heart rate) or multiply by 0.8 for the higher end (80 percent of your maximum heart rate). For example, for a thirty-five-year-old individual:

$$220 - 35 = 185 \times 0.6 = 111; 220 - 35 = 185 \times 0.8 = 148$$

This individual's target heart rate would range from 111 beats per minute at the lower end to 148 at the higher end.

It is important to begin at the lower end of your target heart rate range. As your fitness level improves, you can work toward the higher end of your target heart rate range.

AGE	TARGET HEART RATE
20 years	120–160 beats per minute
30 years	114–152 beats per minute
40 years	108–144 beats per minute
50 years	102–136 beats per minute
60 years	96–128 beats per minute
70 years	90–120 beats per minute
80 years	84–112 beats per minute

Remember these key factors to help you maximize the results for your workout:

•**Frequency:** three to five times per week (five times is optimal)

•**Duration:** twenty to sixty minutes per day

•**Intensity:** stay within your target heart rate zone for twenty to forty minutes

Anaerobic activities are those that are high in intensity yet short in duration. They raise your heart rate for small amounts of time and promote muscular strength.[9] Examples include football, push-ups, sprinting, and racquetball. It has been shown that a combination of both aerobic and anaerobic training has the most beneficial results. Resistance training, such as weightlifting, is also an important part of any exercise program, as it builds muscle and increases strength.

Exercise and building muscle elevate metabolism. You can burn 35 to 50 more calories per day for each pound of muscle gained.[10] When metabolism is raised through exercise, the rise is maintained even hours after your workout is finished. Therefore, fit individuals burn substantial amounts of calories even during a resting state. Because metabolism slows as we age, it is imperative that exercise become an integral part of weight management during the later years of life.

Certified personal trainer Clark Evans provides the following workout chart and tips for the followers of the Nantucket Diet.

CATEGORY	EXERCISE TYPE	FREQUENCY	INTENSITY	TIME
BEGINNER	swimming, stationary bike, mild stair climbing, walking, treadmill walking, most any exercise	3–5 days per week	low to moderate	20 to 60 minutes
INTERMEDIATE	jogging, aerobics, stair climbing, treadmill walking (incline)	4–6 days per week	moderate to moderately high	30 to 60 minutes
ADVANCED	jogging, aerobics, stair climbing, treadmill walking (incline) supplement with weight training	4–6 days per week	high once sufficiently capable	30 to 60 minutes or more

A means of determining if a person's exercise training is primarily aerobic involves talking to the individual while he or she is training. If the individual is able to maintain at least a short conversation, the exercise is primarily aerobic in nature and the individual is most likely not overstressing the body.

If you exercise regularly and eat well but still cannot seem to lose those last few extra pounds, you have reached a plateau. You shouldn't stress about it. Don't weigh yourself too frequently. There are days when you simply retain fluid and weigh a pound or two more than you did the day before. The scale can be deceptive, and you don't want to get discouraged. Even if you lose several pounds rather quickly in the beginning of your weight loss program, the closer you get to reaching your goal, the more difficult it may become to achieve your target weight loss. For those of you lifting weights, your muscles become more developed and therefore you have increased lean body mass; muscle weighs more than fat, so your weight may not be the best indicator of your progress. A better way to judge whether you are slimming down is by monitoring the way your clothes fit. If necessary, increase the length of your workouts and/or the intensity of your workouts. Vary the types of exercise you incorporate into your workouts as well.

EXERCISE IS FOR EVERYONE

Consult your physician before starting an exercise program. If you suffer from heart, lung, or orthopedic problems, or if you have been quite inactive for a long time your doctor may want you to come in for an evaluation. Unless you have serious health concerns, exercise really is for everyone. There are significant benefits for men and women of all ages and races. According to the National Institutes of Health, obesity in children is now at an epidemic rate in the United States.[11] Children who are overweight are at much greater risk for asthma, diabetes, high blood pressure, heart disease, and orthopedic problems. They also may suffer from low self-esteem and depression due to their size. As many as 70 percent of overweight children may become overweight adults.[12] For the first time in history, the average child may not live as long as his or her parents.[13] Therefore, it is imperative that children and adolescents are given the chance to become healthy adults. I was overweight as a child but changing my eating habits and lifestyle has enabled me to remain at a healthy weight into my adulthood. The earlier one begins to establish a healthy lifestyle, the easier it is to maintain in later years. Parents should establish guidelines when it comes to eating and exercise. Teaching children about nutrition is important and keeping them moving is essential.

Statistics show that nearly half of our young people from age twelve to twenty-one are not physically active on a consistent basis and that activity declines dramatically during adolescence.[14] Females are much less physically active than males. Mandatory physical education classes have been declining in school systems over recent years. Enrollment in high school physical education classes has declined from 42 percent in

1991 to 29 percent over the last decade.[15] In response the Surgeon General's office calls on schools to provide daily physical education classes for all grades.[16]

Getting young people interested in school sports and enrolling them in classes such as dance and gymnastics, as well as setting up lessons for swimming, skating, and the like, will help them stay physically fit. Making sure that children and teens remain active inside and outside of school is critical. Family activities such as walking and biking trips, engaging in household chores together, and even taking children with you to the gym are all ways to ensure that your child is developing a healthy exercise pattern.

Adolescents have become increasingly more sedentary because of the amount of time that they spend watching television or playing video games—three to five hours per day, according to many surveys.[17] Sitting in front of the computer is another form of entertainment that has taken over the lifestyles of our young people. Limitations should be placed on these activities and some type of exercise introduced instead. Parents are role models. Children who see their parents making exercise a daily habit are more likely to incorporate exercise into their lives as well.

OLDER ADULTS

The U.S. Surgeon General has found that all people can be helped by moderate levels of activity.[18] In surveys of people age fifty-five or older, 38 percent reported essentially sedentary lifestyles.[19] The National Institute on Aging has found that regular exercise and physical activity are very important to the health and abilities of older adults. Studies have shown that it is beneficial to older individuals to remain as active as they possibly can.[20] As with all exercise programs, it is important to check with your doctor before starting, but for most, the gains far outweigh any potential risk.

Seniors who keep moving increase their strength, flexibility, and clarity of mind. Many elderly people report feeling younger when they engage in some sort of exercise and staying in shape will help them maintain their independence. They also gain a sense of autonomy when able to do things on their own. Sustaining a level of physical fitness as we age will help to prevent a variety of diseases and disabilities.

The older population can greatly benefit from walking. It is low-impact yet has several important health benefits. Enrolling in exercise programs specifically designed for seniors is another option. Swimming is a great choice as well. Everyday household tasks such as cleaning and gardening can also be helpful. Whatever type of activity you select, research has proven that exercise at every age level has remarkable positive effects.

MEN AND WOMEN

There are some differences between men and women when it comes to exercise. Men are apt to exercise more frequently and at elevated intensities.[21] They have less difficulty losing weight than women. Females usually have a lower resting metabolic rate (RMR). Studies show that those with a lower RMR are more prone to gain weight.[22] Women are more likely to store fat in their hips, buttocks, and lower abdomen, while men tend to store fat in their abdominal cavity. Unlike males, females usually do not dramatically increase their size from strength training and so do not need to worry about bulking up from weightlifting programs. Increases in muscle mass are higher in males, while reductions in body fat tend to be slightly higher in females.[23] Both sexes can develop their strength level at the same rate.

Most men work out to build muscle and stay toned. Women typically engage in fitness routines for weight loss. Whatever the differences are when it comes to men and women, why or how they exercise does not matter. The most important factor is that both men and women reap the benefits of staying in shape, especially regarding reduction in the risk of diabetes, heart disease, high blood pressure, elevated cholesterol levels, osteoporosis, and arthritis.

Researchers from Duke University studied the benefits of exercise and diet on overweight men and women with high blood pressure.[24] They compared three groups: those in a diet and exercise program, those in an exercise program alone, and a control group. The group in the diet and exercise program had the best results in terms of lowering blood pressure. This group also demonstrated the best results in terms of lower blood sugar.

Studies have been conducted to evaluate the effects of exercise on lowering cholesterol in men and women. Most research has been consistent in its findings: exercise has a modest effect on lowering total and LDL cholesterol but an important effect on raising HDL cholesterol. This latter benefit has been particularly demonstrated in women.

THE NANTUCKET DIET WORKOUT

Nantucket is one of the most beautiful places in the world. Exercising on the island is a true pleasure for the senses. Whether the sounds of the ocean's mighty waves captures your attention as you walk along Nantucket's one hundred miles of shoreline or the scent of honeysuckle overcomes you as you ride down one of the island's many cycling paths, the offerings of a destination filled with so much natural beauty make an outdoor workout a truly enjoyable experience.

Nantucket provides many kinds of exercise options. Some of these include swimming, surfing, walking, jogging, biking, in-line skating, kayaking, beach volleyball, windsurfing, water skiing, skating, tennis, and golf.

Exercise is one of the cornerstones of the Nantucket Diet. It is a misleading notion that a diet without exercise will offer lifelong cardiovascular and health benefits. Perhaps this is a sobering fact for some, but it should not be. Exercise and diet go hand in hand as part of a comprehensive philosophy for healthy living. Rather than being arduous and restrictive, the exercise and diet program as recommended by the Nantucket Diet should be rewarding and fun.

The following maps of the island show several of the exercise locations for biking, walking, etc. and the number of miles from point to point. For any exercise you choose, you can easily determine the number of calories used during your workout. Whether exercising on Nantucket or in any other location, learning to calculate the number of calories that you burn will be a useful tool in accelerating weight loss.

BICYCLING ON NANTUCKET

One of the best ways to tour Nantucket is by bicycle. The island is only 14 miles long by 3.5 miles wide, and a dedicated cyclist can bike around the entire island in a day. More leisurely trips can be made from town to several beaches, to the village of 'Sconset on the eastern shore, and Madaket on the island's western tip.

1. **SURFSIDE BIKE PATH:** Approximately 2.2 miles along flat terrain.

2. **MILESTONE BIKE PATH:**   Approximately 6 miles with gentle hills.

3. **CLIFF ROAD BIKE PATH:**   Approximately 1.2 miles with rolling terrain.

4. **EEL POINT/DIONIS BEACH BIKE PATH:**   Approximately 0.9 miles with gentle hills.

5. **MADAKET BIKE PATH:**   Approximately 5.5 miles with gentle hills and a winding terrain.

6. **POLPIS BIKE PATH:**   Approximately 8 miles with various size hills and a winding terrain.

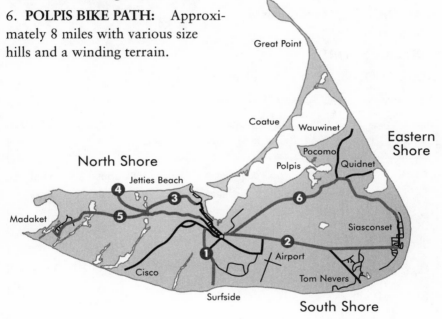

PUBLIC BEACHES

NORTH SHORE

1. **JETTIES BEACH:**   Easy bike ride from town.

2. **BRANT POINT:**   Easy walk or bike ride.

3. **CHILDREN'S BEACH:**   On the harbor, an easy walk from town.

4. **DIONIS:**   Three miles by bike.

5. **FRANCIS STREET BEACH:**   Five-minute walk from Main Street.

SOUTH SHORE

6. SURFSIDE: Located at the end of Surfside Road.

7. MIACOMET: Located at the end of Miacomet Road.

8. CISCO: Four-mile bike ride to the end of Hummock Pond Road.

9. MADAKET: As far west as you can go.

EASTERN SHORE

10. SIASCONSET: 6-mile ride on paved bike path.

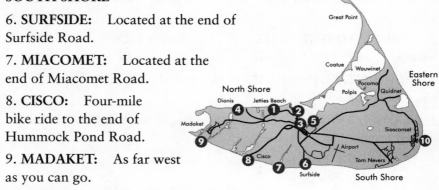

Map information courtesy of Nantucket Island Chamber of Commerce, Copyright.

	GREAT BEACH WALKING LOCATIONS		
Beach	**Approximate Distance**	**Calories Burned**	**Total Time**
Madaket to Cisco	3 miles	675	90 min.
Cisco to Miacomet	2 miles	412	55 min.
Miacomet to Surfside	1⅓ miles	300	40 min.
Surfside to Nobadeer	⅔ mile	150	20 min.
Nobadeer to Madaquecham	2 miles	412	55 min.
Madaquecham to Tom Nevers	3 miles	675	90 min.
Tom Nevers to Siasconset	2½ miles	525	70 min.
Steps to Jetties	½ mile	112	15 min.

The following chart lists a variety of activities and an estimate of the amount of calories burned. The chart is based on an individual weighing 140 pounds.

To figure out the number of calories that you will burn when engaging in a particular activity, add or subtract 10 percent of the listed calories for each 14 pounds above or below 140.[25] Remember the more you weigh, the more energy you expend. For example, someone who weighs 140 pounds and runs at 5 mph for one hour will burn 507 calories, while an individual who weighs 210 pounds will burn 762 calories.

The percentage of calories from fat that are burned is approximately one-third of the total number of calories. For example, if you burn 350 calories in an hour, about 112 of these are derived from fat.

ACTIVITY	CALORIES BURNED PER HOUR
Aerobics, general	380
Aerobics, high impact	444
Aerobics, low impact	317
Badminton, general	285
Baseball	317
Basketball, game	507
Bicycling, low speed	253
Bicycling, high speed	1,014
Bicycling, mountain	538
Bicycling, stationary, high intensity	665
Bicycling, stationary, light intensity	348
Bicycling, stationary, moderate intensity	444
Billiards	159
Bowling	190
Boxing	760
Boxing, punching bag	380
Calisthenics, sit-ups, push-ups, etc., moderate effort	286
Calisthenics, vigorous effort	507
Canoeing or rowing, intense effort	760
Canoeing or rowing, light effort	190
Canoeing or rowing, moderate effort	444
Carpentry	222
Child care, dressing, feeding, etc.	221
Circuit training	507
Cleaning, heavy	286
Cleaning, light to moderate	159
Coaching, sports	253
Construction, general	349

ACTIVITY	CALORIES BURNED PER HOUR
Cooking	159
Cricket	317
Croquet	159
Dancing, ballet, aerobic, modern	380
Dancing, ballroom	286
Darts	286
Diving, off board	190
Electrical work, plumbing	222
Elliptical trainer, general	605
Farming	349
Fencing	380
Fishing from boat, sitting	159
Fishing, ice, sitting	127
Fishing in water with waders	380
Fishing, standing from beach or pond	222
Football, competitive	570
Football, touch	507
Frisbee	190
Gardening	317
Golf	253
Golf, carrying golf bag	306
Golf, miniature or driving range	190
Gymnastics	253
Hacky sack	253
Handball	760
Health club exercise	349
Hiking	453
Hockey, field	507
Hockey, ice	507
Horse grooming	380
Horse racing	507
Horseback riding, trotting	412
Horseback riding, walking	159
Hunting	317
Jet skiing	403
Jogging	444

ACTIVITY	CALORIES BURNED PER HOUR
Karate, kickboxing, judo, etc.	634
Kayaking	317
Kickball	444
Lacrosse	507
Moving, lifting, carrying heavy items	507
Mowing lawn, riding	159
Mowing lawn, walking	349
Music playing, drums or standing in band	253
Music playing, sitting at piano, guitar, violin, cello, etc.	154
Paddleboat	253
Painting, wallpapering, etc.	286
Pilates, intense	373
Pilates, light to moderate	280
Ping-Pong	253
Polo	507
Pushing or pulling baby stroller	320
Racquetball	444
Raking	253
Reading	72
Rock climbing	700
Roller skating, in-line skating	444
Rope jumping	634
Rowing, stationary	603
Rugby	634
Running, 5 mph	507
6 mph	634
7 mph	729
8 mph	855
9 mph	951
10 mph	1,014
Running up stairs	951
Sailing	220
Sailing, competitive	317
Scrubbing floors	343
Scuba diving	444
Shoveling snow	380

ACTIVITY	CALORIES BURNED PER HOUR
Shuffleboard	190
Skateboarding	317
Skating, ice	444
Skating, speed	951
Ski machine	603
Skiing, cross country, high intensity	570
Skiing, cross country, moderate intensity	507
Skiing, cross country, uphill	1,045
Skiing, downhill, high intensity, racing	507
Skiing, downhill, moderate intensity	380
Ski jumping	444
Sledding, tobogganing, etc.	444
Sleeping	45
Snorkeling	317
Snowmobiling	222
Snowshoeing	507
Soccer, competitive	634
Soccer, general	444
Softball	317
Squash	760
Stair machine	400
Stretching	253
Surfing, body or board	390
Swimming, butterfly	697
Swimming, moderate intensity, backstroke, sidestroke	507
Swimming, treading water, moderate intensity	253
Swimming, vigorous intensity, breaststroke, treading water	634
Tennis, doubles	380
Tennis, singles	507
Volleyball, beach	507
Volleyball, gym	253
Walk/run, playing with child	306
Walking, 2 mph	200
3 mph	300
4 mph	400
Walking 3 mph uphill	420

ACTIVITY	CALORIES BURNED PER HOUR
Walking on beach	450
Walking upstairs or on high-incline treadmill	563
Wallyball	253
Water aerobics	253
Water polo	634
Waterskiing	444
Water volleyball	190
Weightlifting, heavy	380
Weightlifting, moderate	190
Whitewater rafting	317
Windsurfing	400
Yoga, intense or power (ashtanga)	430
Yoga, low to moderate intensity (hatha, etc.)	254

REFERENCES

Chapter 1

1. Konner, M. *The Tangled Wing,* Harper and Row, 1982: 5–7.
2. Konner, M. *The Tangled Wing,* Harper and Row, 1982: 370.
3. Nestle, M. *Science,* February 7, 2003, 299(5608): 781.
4. Willett, W. et al. *NEJM,* August 5, 1999, 341(6): 427.
5. www.who.int/whr/2002/en/. November 7, 2004.
6. Pinhas-Hamiel, O. et al. *J. Pediatr.,* May 1996, 128(5 Pt 1):591.
7. American Association of Clinical Endocrinologists/American College of Endocrinology Obesity Position Statement; 1998 Revision: 4.
8. Willett, W. et al. *NEJM,* August 5, 1999, 341(6): 427.
9. National Heart, Lung, and Blood Institute. Clinical Guidelines on the Identification, Evaluation and Treatment of Overweight and Obesity in Adults, 1998: 94.
10. Ibid., xiv.
11. Flegal, K. et al. *JAMA,* October 9, 2002, 288(14): 1723.
12. Sturm R. *Arch. Intern. Med.,* October 13, 2003, 163(18): 2146.
13. Hill, J. et al. *Science,* Feb 7, 2003, 299(5608): 853.
14. Ogden, C. et al. *JAMA,* October 9, 2002, 288(14): 1728. Strauss, R. et al. *JAMA,* December 12, 2001, 286(22): 2845.
15. Booth, M. et al. *Am. J. Clin. Nutr.,* January 2003, 77(1): 29–36.
16. Fontaine, K.R. et al. *JAMA,* January 8, 2003, 289(2): 187.
17. Mokdad, A. et al. *JAMA,* March 10, 2004, 291(10): 1238.
18. Wolf, A. et al. *Obesity Research,* March 1998, 6(2): 97.
19. Puhl, R. et al. *Obesity Research,* December 2001, 9(12): 788. Strauss, R.S. *Arch. Pediatr. Adolesc. Med.,* August 2003, 157(8): 746.
20. Schwartz, M. et al. *Obesity Research,* September 2003, 11(9): 1033.
21. Diabetes Prevention Program Research Group. *NEJM,* February 7, 2002, 346(6): 393.
22. Rosenbaum, M. et al. *NEJM,* August 7, 1997, 337(6): 396.
23. National Heart, Lung, and Blood Institute. Clinical Guidelines on the Identification, Evaluation and Treatment of Overweight and Obesity in Adults, 1998: 68.
24. Ibid.
25. Hill, J. et al. *Science,* February 7, 2003, 299(5608): 853.
26. Halford, J.C. et al. *Obesity Research,* January 2004, 12(1): 171.
27. Robinson, T.N. *JAMA,* October 27, 1999, 282(16): 1561.

28. Critser, G. "Measuring Up: New Front Line in the Battle of the Bulge." *New York Times,* May 18, 2003.
29. Rozin, P. et al. *Psychol. Sci.,* September 2003, 14(5): 450.
30. Hill, J. et al. *Science,* February 7, 2003, 299(5608): 853.
31. Manson, J. et al. *Arch. Intern. Med.,* February 9, 2004, 164: 249.
32. Mokdad, A. *JAMA,* March 10, 2004, 291(10): 1238.
33. msnbc.msn.com/id/4500530, March 10, 2004.
34. Drewnowski, A. *Am. J. Clin. Nutr.,* January 2004, 79(1): 6.

Chapter 2

1. Foster, G. et al. *NEJM,* May 22, 2003, 348(21): 2082.
2. Freedman, M. et al. *Obesity Research,* 2001, 9: 1S.
3. Bravata, D. et al. *JAMA,* April 9, 2003, 289(14): 1837.
4. Golay, A. *Am. J. Clin. Nutr.,* February 1996, 63(2): 174.
5. Stern, L. et al. *Ann. Int. Med.,* May 18, 2004, 140(10): 778.
6. Freedman, M. et al. *Obesity Research,* 2001, 9: 1S, 4S.
7. Reddy, S.T. *Am. J. Kidney. Dis.,* August 2002, 40(2): 265–74.
8. Choi, H. *NEJM,* March 11, 2004, 350(11): 1093.
9. web.mit.edu/newsoffice/2004/carbs.html, November 7, 2004.
10. www.msnbc.com/news/991292.asp, November 15, 2003.
11. USDA Coordinated Nutrition Research Program on Health and Nutrition; Effects of Popular Weight Loss Diets, January 10, 2001.
12. Freedman, M. et al. *Obesity Research,* 2001, 9: 1S.
13. Mela, D. *Obesity Research,* 2001, 9: S249.
14. www.lifespan.org/services/bmed/wt_loss/nwcr/, November 7, 2004.
15. Klem, M. et al. *Am. J. Clin. Nutr.,* 1997, 66: 239.
16. Shick, S. et al. *J. Am. Diet. Assn.,* 1998, 98: 408.
17. McGuire, M. et al. *J. Consult. Clin. Psych.,* 1999, 67: 177.
18. Klem, M. et al. *Am. J. Clin. Nutr.,* 1997, 66: 239.
19. Ibid.
20. Klem, M. et al. *Obesity Research,* 2000, 8: 438.

Chapter 3

1. Joseph, A. *J. Am. Coll. Cardiol.,* August 1993, 22(2): 459.
2. Menotti, A. *Eur. J. Epidemiology,* July 1999, 15(6): 507.
3. Campbell, T. et al. *The American Journal of Cardiology,* Nov. 26, 1998, 82(10) supplement 2:18.
4. Rastogi, T. *Am. J. Clin. Nutr.,* April 2004, 79(4): 582.
5. Ornish, D. et al. *JAMA,* December 16, 1998, 280(23): 2001.
6. Wolk, A. et al. *JAMA,* June 2, 1999, 281(21): 1998.

7. www.iom.edu/report.asp?id=5519, November 7, 2004.
8. www.iom.edu/report.asp?id=4340, November 7, 2004.
9. www.americanheart.org/presenter.jhtml?identifier=4574, November 7, 2004.
10. www.americanheart.org/presenter.jhtml?identifier=4627, November 7, 2004.
11. Hu, F. *JAMA,* November 27, 2002, 288(20): 2568.
12. Trichopoulou, A. *NEJM,* June 26, 2003, 348(26): 2599.
13. http://www.hsph.harvard.edu/nutritionsource/pyramids.html, November 7, 2004.
14. http://www.health.gov/dietaryguidelines/dga2005/AgendaPublicJan2004Mtg.pdf, November 7, 2004.
15. Lieber, C. *Cleveland Clin. J. Med.,* November 2003, 70(11): 945.
16. www.americanheart.org/presenter.jhtml?identifier=1330, November 7, 2004.
17. www.americanheart.org/presenter.jhtml?identifier=4452, November 7, 2004.
18. Yusuf, S. *NEJM,* January 2000, 342(3): 154. Lonn, E. *Diab. Care,* November 2002, 25(11): 1919.
19. Heart Protection Study Collaborative Group; *Lancet,* July 2002, 360 (9326): 23.
20. Levy, A. *Diab. Care,* 2004, 27: 925.
21. Harris, W.S. *Cleveland Clin. J. Med.,* March 2004, 71(3): 208.
22. Ibid.
23. www.americanheart.org/presenter.jhtml?identifier=3006581, November 7, 2004.
24. Pittler, M. *Am. J. Clin. Nutr.,* April 2004, 79(4): 529.

Chapter 4

1. DIGAMI Study Group; Malmberg, K. *JACC,* July 1995, 26(1): 57. Van den Berghe, G. et al. *NEJM,* November 8, 2001, 345(19): 1359.
2. Lakka, H. *JAMA,* December 4, 2002, 288(21): 2709.
3. ADA Clinical Practice Recommendations 2004, *Diab. Care,* January 2004, S1: s9.
4. Diabetes Prevention Program Research Group. *NEJM,* February 7, 2002, 346(6): 393.
5. Ludwig, D. et al. *Pediatrics,* March 1999, 103(3): e26.
6. UKPDS 34, *Lancet,* September 12, 1998, 352: 854.

Chapter 5

1. Brewer, E. *Eat. Behav.,* August 2003, 4(2): 159–71.
2. Wadden, T. *Endocr. Metab. Clin.,* December 2003, 32(4).
3. Ibid.
4. Ibid.
5. Ibid.
6. Wing, R. *Primary Care Clinics in Office Practice,* June 2003, 30(2).

7. Ibid.
8. Gillman, M.W. *Arch. Fam. Medicine,* March 2000, 9(3): 235.
9. Freedman, M. et al. *Obesity Research,* 2001, 9:1S.
10. National Heart, Lung, and Blood Institute. Clinical Guidelines on the Identification, Evaluation and Treatment of Overweight and Obesity in Adults, 1998.
11. Ibid.: 77, 79.
12. Freedman, M. et al. *Obesity Research,* 2001, 9:1S.
13. Levine, J. *Am. J. Clin. Nutr.,* December 2000, 72(6): 1451.
14. National Heart, Lung, and Blood Institute. Clinical Guidelines on the Identification, Evaluation and Treatment of Overweight and Obesity in Adults, 1998: 78.
15. Ibid.: 70.

Chapter 6

1. www.naaso.com/news/, October 13, 2003.
2. Tuomilehto, J. et al. *JAMA,* March 10, 2004, 291(10): 1213.
3. Prentice, A.M. *Obesity Rev.,* November 2003, 4(4): 187.
4. Katan, M.B. et al. *Mayo Clin. Proc.,* August 2001, 78(8): 965.
5. Talbot, L.A. *J. Am. Geriatr. Soc.,* March 2003, 51(3): 387.
6. Harris, J.A., Benedict F.G. A Biometric Study of the Basal Metabolism of Man, Washington DC, Carnegie Institute, 1919, no. 279.
7. Frankenfield, D. et al. *J. Am. Diet. Assn.,* April 1998, 98(4): 439.
8. Shetty, P.S. et al. *Eur. J. Clin. Nutr.,* February 1996, 50(Suppl 1): S11.
9. Frankenfield, D. et al. *J. Am. Diet. Assn.,* April 1998, 98(4): 439.
10. www.unu.edu/unupress/food2/uid01e/uid01e02.htm, November 14, 2004.
11. http://books.nap.edu/books/0309085373/html/131.html, November 14, 2004.
12. Shetty, P.S. et al. *Eur. J. Clin. Nutr.,* February 1996, 50(Suppl 1): S11.

Chapter 7

1. National Heart, Lung, and Blood Institute. Clinical Guidelines on the Identification, Evaluation and Treatment of Overweight and Obesity in Adults, 1998.
2. Champagne C.M. *J. Am. Diet. Assn.,* October 2002, 102(10): 1428.

Chapter 8

1. http://my.webmd.com/content/article/46/2731_1661.htm, Controlling How Much You Eat, Article 46/2731-1661, March 20, 2004.
2. www.uwlax.edu, Predicting Proper Portion Sizes, March 20, 2004.

Chapter 9

1. http://my.webmd.com/content/article/46/2731_1661.htm, Controlling How Much You Eat, Article 46/2731-1661, March 20, 2004.

Chapter 10

1. http://www.americanheart.org/presenter.jhtml?identifier=820, Physical Activity and Cardiovascular Health Fact Sheet, January 13, 2004.
2. Ibid.
3. http://www.primusweb.com/fitnesspartner/library/activity/motomove.htm, The Motivation to Move, Vicki R. Pierson and Renee Cloe.
4. Ibid.
5. http://www.americanheart.org/presenter.jhtml?identifier=820, Physical Activity and Cardiovascular Health Fact Sheet, January 2004.
6. http://www.inq7.net/lif/2004/mar/30/lif_21-1.htm, You May Not Be Losing Pounds but Inches, March 30, 2004.
7. http://www.freeweightlosscenter.com/article13.htm, Article 13, Aerobic or Anaerobic, November 17, 2003.
8. http://www.nhlbi.nih.gov/health/public/heart/other/hdw_act.pdf, Physical Activity and Heart Disease, December 2003.
9. http://atozfitness.healthology.com/focus_article.asp?f=men_fitness&c=maximize_aerobicworkout#Definition%20of%20Aerobic, The Iron Connection Glossary of Fitness, November 17, 2003.
10. http://www.foxfitnesstraining.com/SomeFactsWomenandStrengthTraining.html, Exercise in the Privacy and Comfort of Your Own Home; Conditioning Research, 2002; 16(4): 645–48.
11. http://www.nih.gov/news/WordonHealth/jun2002/childhoodobesity.htm, Childhood Obesity on the Rise, June 2002.
12. Ibid.
13. http://www.epolitix.com/EN/ForumBriefs/200312/F287E1A5-672D-4A6E-A669-3A4AB1C9D7DB.htm, Forum Brief: Obesity—Wanless Report, December 9, 2003.
14. http://www.nih.gov/news/WordonHealth/jun2002/childhoodobesity.htm, Childhood Obesity on the Rise, June 2002.
15. http://www.americanheart.org/presenter.jhtml?identifier=820, Physical Activity and Cardiovascular Health Fact Sheet, January 13, 2004.
16. http://www.nih.gov/news/WordonHealth/jun2002/childhoodobesity.htm, Childhood Obesity on the Rise, June 2002.
17. Ibid.
18. http://www.nia.nih.gov/exercisebook/chapter1.htm, What Can Exercise Do for Me?, National Institute on Aging, January 10, 2004.

19. http://www.americanheart.org/presenter.jhtml?identifier=820, Physical Activity and Cardiovascular Health Fact Sheet. January 13, 2004.
20. http://www.nia.nih.gov/exercisebook/chapter1.htm, What Can Exercise Do for Me?, National Institute on Aging, January 10, 2004.
21. http://www.abfabfitness.com/exercise_and_women.html, Exercise and Women, January 12, 2004.
22. Ibid.
23. Ibid.
24. www.infoaging.org, Exercise Information Center, December 2003.
25. *Allan Borushek's Calorie and Fat Counter.* Costa Mesa, CA, Allan Borushek and Assoc. Inc., 1991.

INDEX

ABOUT THE AUTHORS

SOL JACOBS, M.D. practices endocrinology in the greater Boston area. Dr. Jacobs is a Fellow of the American College of Endocrinology and is a faculty member of Tufts University School of Medicine.

JANE CONWAY CASPE is a fashion model working and living in the greater Boston area and on Nantucket. She is a fourth-generation descendant of one of the original settling families of the island of Nantucket.